WONDERFUL AND WEIRD

Thumbnail Sketches from a Career in Psychiatric Nursing

MALCOLM KING, RN; MS; CS

authorHOUSE

AuthorHouse™
1663 Liberty Drive
Bloomington, IN 47403
www.authorhouse.com
Phone: 1 (800) 839-8640

© 2018 Malcolm King, RN; MS; CS. All rights reserved.

No part of this book may be reproduced, stored in a retrieval system, or transmitted by any means without the written permission of the author.

Published by AuthorHouse 03/09/2018

ISBN: 978-1-5462-3282-7 (sc)
ISBN: 978-1-5462-3280-3 (hc)
ISBN: 978-1-5462-3281-0 (e)

Library of Congress Control Number: 2018903090

Print information available on the last page.

Any people depicted in stock imagery provided by Getty Images are models, and such images are being used for illustrative purposes only.
Certain stock imagery © Getty Images.

This book is printed on acid-free paper.

Because of the dynamic nature of the Internet, any web addresses or links contained in this book may have changed since publication and may no longer be valid. The views expressed in this work are solely those of the author and do not necessarily reflect the views of the publisher, and the publisher hereby disclaims any responsibility for them.

To psych nurses everywhere, who love
their wonderful and weird work.

Introduction

Probably every nurse in the world has, at one time, muttered to himself or herself, in the middle of some impossibly wild shift, "I should write a book about this stuff!" This would then be inevitably be followed by a shrug of the shoulders and the next thought: "But no one would believe it!" Because nursing is a profession in which you see things that others who are not nurses just wouldn't ever see, or even imagine as being possible.

There are many other occupations in which workers are constantly interacting with the general public, and they will all have their weird and wonderful stories to tell after a few years, of course. But other than the experiences of first responders, there really is little to equal the intensity of the interactions between nurses and their patients. For in nursing we see these folks in unusually vulnerable and desperate situations, and all general hospital nurses, whether they work in emergency rooms, intensive care units, or on regular medical-surgical units, soon have stores of horrific, incredible, and inspiring tales with which to regale each other during those tough shifts.

Psychiatric nursing certainly has a rich share of such tales, perhaps even more so due to psychiatry's unique place among the various branches of medicine, for psychiatry does have three crucial aspects that the other branches don't.

Firstly, psychiatric disorders simply hold a unique fascination for many people that physical illnesses do not have, as historically we have had such difficulty in explaining what they are, what causes them, and how to treat them. On occasions, the strange behaviors often associated with mental illness have been interpreted as indicating positive gifts from the gods, but more often they have been viewed more as indicating the presence of evil. Over the centuries, humanity has been fascinated by mental illness, sometimes healthily so, but more often morbidly so.

At a personal level, from an early age we may be warned by our exasperated mothers that we will be sent to the local psychiatric hospital if we don't behave properly, and we wonder to ourselves what must be going on there. As adults there's a good probability that we know family members, friends, or neighbors who have suffered with suicidality or other mental illnesses. When I was eight years old, my family moved to a new house, soon to be told by a neighbor that a previous owner had hung himself in that house. I was too young to understand exactly what that meant, but I was aware that my parents were uncomfortable talking about the story, and consequently I always remembered it. Many people have similar sorts of stories. Plus, every now and then we see on TV some horrific mass killing by someone diagnosed with a mental illness.

So, through our lives, we develop a curiosity about—and usually a fear of—psychiatry and mental illness.

Secondly, psychiatric nurses routinely work with severely ill people who adamantly deny that they have any illness at all. True, people experiencing the first symptoms of a heart attack may deny that these symptoms are due to their actually having the heart attack, but that is usually more just hoping for the best than real denial, and as soon as the heart attack is confirmed, patients quickly acknowledges their need for medical help, and are very grateful when that help comes.

But patients with major mental illness such as schizophrenia will often deny that anything is really wrong with them their entire lives. No matter how many times they are admitted to hospital, or even jail, due to behaviors associated with that illness, they will often steadfastly maintain that denial. That denial then may lead to noncompliance with prescribed psychiatric medications, which leads in turn to the illness never being controlled except when they are in hospital and have to take medications.

Thirdly, psychiatry historically has often appeared to be more like a social or political science than a medical science. This has resulted in many members of the public, as well as many nurses and doctors in the other branches of medicine, being openly skeptical as to whether psychiatry should even be counted as a medical science at all. Psychiatric nurses, therefore, often find themselves on the defensive regarding the legitimacy of the foundations of their practices.

Psychiatry has always been an unstable and inexact science and has become oddly prone to the development of theories that seem to mirror the political themes of particular social eras. For instance, the political-social pendulum swings endlessly from right to left, and in my lifetime, the swing of this pendulum has coincided with quite different beliefs in psychiatry about what causes mental illnesses and what the best treatment for them might be.

This is really just a version of the old nature versus nurture debate about what is most influential in shaping human behaviors: is it the society that we grow up in (including our families) or our inherently biological being (the result of our evolution).

Thus, in a liberal, left-wing political period, free-enterprise capitalism is seen by many people as responsible for all of the problems of mankind, including mental illness. In this theory, the causes for human problems do not lie with individuals themselves; rather, it lies with the greater society, which is seen as being oppressive. And in this society, parents, particularly mothers, sometimes replicate the oppressive strategies of the society that they live in, and then end up rearing schizophrenic children.

The political decades of the 1960s and 1970s were predominantly left-wing, and the psychiatric theories of this period—the time I started in psychiatric nursing—mirrored that political narrative.

Variations along the theme of: 'Insanity is the only sane reaction to an insane society,' were the cry of radical psychiatrists such as Thomas Szasz in the US (1) and those at the Tavistock Clinic in the UK, and that found a distinct echo in psychiatric theory.

For to many people in the profession and others involved in left-wing politics, mental illness was viewed as being entirely due to capitalism and as something that would inevitably simply wither away once a socialist society had been established.

Although psychiatric medications were routinely given to patients (new antipsychotic, antidepressant, and mood stabilizers were regularly coming onto the market by then), medications were viewed by purists as being of limited curative value, with the only real long-term answer to mental illness lying in helping patients gain insight through psychodynamic individual, group, or milieu therapy (or a combination of these) into the distortions of their thinking and emotions imposed upon them by society.

With inpatient psychiatry, the "therapeutic community" was seen as being the real curative factor, as it would free the patients from the oppression of their real-life communities and thereby correct their previously distorted thinking. The concept of such a therapeutic community went back to post–World War II British egalitarianism, with psychiatric units in the 1960s and 1970s consequently being referred to as "therapeutic milieus."

The 1980s then gradually ushered in a more conservative, right-wing political era, with the focus more on individuals being responsible for their own lives through the decisions that they make, rather than attributing all of their problems to society.

This eventually became mirrored in psychiatric theory by an emphasis on viewing mental illness not as being caused by society as a whole, but as an individual illness, caused by physical, chemical imbalances and often the result of genetic predispositions.

Parents were no longer seen as being potentially "schizophrenogenic" by the way in which they reared their children, but by passing on their schizophrenic genes to them. Psycho-dynamically orientated psychiatry became gradually replaced by the medical-biological model of psychiatry in which a mental illness is seen as having a physical origin within the patient's brain. Mental illness became to be viewed as being absolutely most effectively treated by medications designed to correct the chemical changes going on in the patient's brain.

For, by this time, it was apparent that, no matter how many community meetings patients with major mental illnesses attended, no matter how many therapeutic groups they went to, or how many psychotherapy sessions they had, if they didn't take their psychiatric medications, then everything else was pretty much dust in the wind. These nonmedical treatments, therefore, went pretty quickly from being vital curative factors to being adjunctive therapies that might or might not be helpful.

Psycho-dynamically orientated theories of the earlier decades still often receive lip service, but in real practice they started to fade out from the 1980s onward. For instance, inpatient psychiatric units still commonly refer to themselves as "therapeutic milieus," but that no longer means trying to create an idealistic egalitarian mini society capable of curing mental illness; it is more along the lines of developing a respectful and professional environment that will make it more likely that the patients will not behave in violent ways, and will take their prescribed medications.

In my experience, it is this unstable nature of psychiatric theory that contributes to the hesitation of the general public in accepting psychiatry as a genuinely scientific branch of medicine. The different theories tend to come and go as the political pendulum swings, and this happens in a manner simply not seen in the other medical branches.

And that means that, in a given era, the treatment of patients is not necessarily based on medical science. It's sobering for me to look back and see that, for years, my psychiatric nursing practice was based at least in part on political and social theory, not scientific medical theory.

And, unfortunately, when you've got the wrong theory, it's not just a theoretical matter because real patients are involved; it becomes a practical and ethical matter. You can then end up harming patients rather than helping them, as some of my clinical sketches sadly show (for example, Sketches # 14 and 15).

My hope is that research-based biological psychiatry will end up definitively proving to the doubters that we are, indeed, a legitimate branch of medical science rather than a social science, and that our past politically based flip-flops will cease. But only time will tell that!

Meanwhile, these different social, political, and psychiatric theories were directly reflected in various concrete aspects of psychiatric nursing practice. When I started psychiatric nursing in 1971 in England, male nurses wore grey suits as uniforms, and the female nurses wore their traditional variously colored starched uniforms. But gradually, over time, we stopped wearing uniforms on the grounds that it emphasized a "power differential" between staff members and patients that was harmful to the effective treatment of patients in the egalitarian therapeutic milieu.

In the therapeutic milieu, we had to replicate what was then desired in our larger society so that patients and staff members would be seen as perfectly equal in status. So psychiatric nurses then started wearing street clothes—mufti as it was called.

When I started nursing, I also wore an identity badge giving my name and professional title, but after a while that was then also deemed to emphasize a power differential between nurses and patients that was unacceptable in an egalitarian community. So, in some settings, we stopped wearing badges, to the frequent torment of visitors who often couldn't tell staff members from patients when they came onto the unit, and would often end up asking patients their questions, in the belief that they were staff members.

Patients rather than staff members were made chairmen of the daily community meetings to make the relationship appear egalitarian, but everyone—patients and staff members alike—knew that this was a sham, done for the sake of appearances, and that the real power was always with the staff members.

When the medical-biological model started to predominate, it became acceptable again for staff members to wear identity badges, to the immense relief of those poor confused visitors. Hospital survey bodies such as the

Joint Commission made it mandatory, actually, in order to provide patients with accurate information about who was caring for them.

Uniforms didn't come back completely, in part because of the potential cost involved for psychiatric hospitals, but these days it is common to see nurses in some form of scrubs uniform in psychiatric settings.

Similarly, in the 1960s and '70s, psychiatric therapeutic milieus were viewed as necessarily having open rather than locked doors. These units were supposed to represent in miniature the ideal greater open society, and locked doors were not part of that narrative. Locked doors would mirror the closed, oppressive society which had caused the mental illness in the first place, and which would therefore be harmful to patients' treatment.

Open doors were also supposed to counter the social stigma of psychiatric patients being associated with violent behaviors and therefore needing to be locked up. Psychiatric units or hospitals with open doors were, in reality, not open at all. Any patient who actually decided to just walk out of that open door was quickly brought back by staff members, forcibly if necessary. But, again, it was the appearance rather than the reality that was important at that time. Any hospital that still had locked units at that time was considered to be a shameful throwback to the asylum era, so a truly modern hospital simply had to have open doors.

But by the 1980s it was no longer possible to deny that, when people with major psychiatric illnesses are in an actively symptomatic phase of their illness, they are indeed more likely than the general population to behave violently, though patients in a stable phase of their illness are not more likely to behave violently. This meant recognizing that patients requiring hospitalization do indeed often present serious safety risks. In the face of this evidence, gradually the theoretically open doors became locked again as hospitals became conscious of these safety risks.

For the psychiatric nurse, the two different epochs presented different rewards and different problems (2/3). The period of psychosocial, psycho-dynamically orientated psychiatry attributed mental illness to family and social stressors, with the inevitable implicit suggestion that the resulting illnesses might be impossible to impact until families or society were changed, and the therapeutic community or milieu provided the model for that required change.

Psychiatric nurses were the only members of the treatment team to be present twenty-four hours a day on this milieu, and they were responsible for organizing and managing it, thus becoming vital members of the team. This model additionally gave psychiatric nurses the rewarding opportunity of considering in detail why patients might be thinking and behaving in their individual manner, and of how nurses might involve themselves in that illness in a human way. Nurses were therefore easily able to feel compassion and empathy in their work, which was very rewarding for them.

The problem was that, no matter what nurses did with patients over months or years, no one really believed that the patients were going to be cured, even if the theory clearly stated that the egalitarian therapeutic milieu was in itself a curative factor.

In this essentially pessimistic view, nurses saw patients as basically being incurable, with the nurses' role being largely to try to bring some meaningful human contact into the patients' lives in an effort to ameliorate as best they could the horror of the illness. So the psychiatric nurse then could feel good about the nature of his/her professional relationship with their patients, while also wishing that what they were doing had a better chance of actually effectively treating the patients' illnesses.

In the era of biological psychiatry, this was turned the other way around. The view of mental illness became a more optimistic one, as in this model the illness was seen as a biochemical, neurological, genetic condition which could ultimately be treated as successfully as medical illnesses could be treated. It was very rewarding for psychiatric nurses to believe that they were part of successfully treating and perhaps even ultimately curing illnesses.

The problem for nurses in this model was that it might lead them to think that all they have to do is to give out medications to their patients and throw in a little patient education. Finding a way to go beyond being simply glorified medication nurses was therefore the challenge for the psychiatric nurses in that era.

While psychiatric nurses may have ultimately felt more hopeful about their patients' illnesses, they also may have been unsure of how to show more of a human touch in their work with those patients. But even now, when no one believes that an egalitarian therapeutic milieu is, by itself, a curative factor for mental illness, it remains essential that psychiatric nurses have the kindness, patience, empathy, milieu management skills, knowledge, and compassion necessary to create a safe, structured, and caring hospital unit—a unit in which patients can feel some degree of trust and confidence in their nurses, and are therefore more likely to behave in safe ways and to voluntarily accept their medication treatment both in hospital and out of it.

It is somewhat paradoxical that, in the era when psychiatric nursing practice was based on pseudo medical science, in some ways nurses felt more certain about their roles than they do now in an era in which their nursing practice is based on real medical science.

This identity crisis isn't unique to nursing, however, as nonmedical professionals who work on psychiatric treatment teams as psychologists and social workers are perhaps even more unsure of how they ultimately fit into the biological-medical model of psychiatry

Perhaps accurately reflecting the instability of psychiatry as a branch of medicine, out of the twelve hospitals that I worked in which were either purely psychiatric or had some psychiatric inpatient units, seven have now closed completely or have closed their inpatient units.

After I retired in 2015, I found myself occasionally thinking back on the incidents in my career that had most baffled, infuriated, delighted, and influenced me, and had meaningfully contributed to my career as a nurse. I wondered if it would be of any value to other psychiatric nurses for me to sketch out these incidents and to add my own thoughts about why I saw them as being important to me.

So I have organized this book as a series of brief sketches, with my thoughts added at the end of each. They are largely arranged in chronological order following the progression of my career, as time line continuity does help make sense of what happened and why. The sketches are a mixture of clinical patient stories, management situations, and educational experiences, along with some historical commentary, and perhaps even some self-indulgent reminiscing.

In order to protect the privacy of patients and staff members referred to in these sketches, I have omitted the actual names of the hospitals that I worked in, and I have changed all of the initials and many of the personal and clinical details of patients and of the incidents they were involved in, as well as those of my colleagues.

My hope is that practicing psychiatric nurses might find some interest and value in reading about the sorts of incidents that they may well be confronted with themselves as they move through their own careers. Also, psychiatric nurse educators may find the clinical sketches in the book useful in their work, as may nurse educators attempting to engage general nursing students doing their dreaded psychiatric rotation.

Looking at these sketches, I see a number of them as involving negative incidents. But perhaps this is just as well, for such incidents do have a motivational side to them in that they oblige us to find a way to prevent them from happening again. Football coaches invariably say it's the games they lost that they remember most vividly, while most of the ones that they won tend to blur together in their minds. Just as the games that the teams lost provide the motivation for the coach to understand and then fix the mistakes that led to the loss, negative clinical incidents can provide that same sort of motivation to psychiatric nurses.

Although I ended up spending more years of my career in management than in clinical positions, the memories I find I hold most clearly and dearly are the clinical ones involving real patients, as it should be for a nurse.

CHAPTER 1

A Hampshire, UK, Hospital

Sketch # 1

I had gone to a Hampshire, UK, university in 1967 to study physiology and biochemistry as my major. When I had to pick a track for my minor study, I had little idea of what to do until an incident occurred in my freshman college dormitory, South Stoneham House. There was a young man there who was clearly "different" from the rest of us. He kept entirely to himself and never talked to anyone unless it was unavoidable. At supper he wouldn't eat any of the regular food; rather, he would take only two slices of bread, sprinkle salt over the slices, and cut the crust off them. He would then eat the crusts and throw away the rest of the bread. Shortly after it had turned dark each evening, he would run around the tennis courts five times, increasing his speed as he went, before going to bed. We mercilessly mocked him in private, but we also knew that what ailed him was completely beyond our ken, and in reality, we were perfectly afraid of him.

After several weeks he simply disappeared, and a few days later we were told by the dormitory staff that he had killed himself.

In an effort to try to find out what on earth had just happened before my eyes, I decided on psychology as my minor course of study.

At the time that I graduated from university, people with a degree in biochemistry usually went to work for a pharmaceutical company. But that just didn't appeal to me at that point, so I was unemployed for a few weeks. Eventually, the exasperated man at the unemployment office told me that there were available nursing assistant positions at a local hospital, and I should do that, "Until your perfect job comes along."

I blithely assumed that this hospital was a normal general hospital dealing with medical and surgical patients, and it came as a great surprise to me when I turned up at their human resources office to discover that it was actually the old county insane asylum founded in 1852, now with a different name.

But, as I had done psychology as my minor course of study at university, and I wasn't looking forward to facing my unemployment officer again, I was soon working at the hospital as a nursing assistant.

Being at the bottom of the staffing heap, I was naturally given the position that no one else would voluntarily take—a rotating day-evening job in the psychogeriatric ward. I expected the worst when I went there because few people held back in confiding to me how awful it was going to be, but I was pleasantly surprised to discover that I actually rather liked it.

One patient there was N. M., a sixty-year-old man with a long history of undifferentiated schizophrenia. He was very obese, with gynecomastia (enlarged breasts) and occasional leakage of milk due to the large doses of chlorpromazine (trade names Thorazine and Largactil) that he had been on for many years. He rarely got out of bed as walking was difficult for him. He also had a speech impediment and had no teeth, making it difficult to understand what he was saying, particularly when he started to talk louder and louder if people couldn't make out what he was saying the first time.

In my twenty-one-year-old life I had never met anyone remotely like him, or even imagined anyone like him could possibly exist, so I ended up spending quite a lot of time with him. I never really did grasp much of what he was saying, and all I ever said to him was routine stuff such as: "Good morning, N. I see that Pompey actually won yesterday! Can I help lift you further up the bed? Can I get you something to drink? The weather's miserable outside." And so on. But, after a while, he would smile a misshapen smile at me when I came over to his bed.

Discovering that my working in a nursing role could actually make a small positive difference in an individual patient's life was oddly perplexing to me. At that age, I had envisioned great advances for mankind were about to take place, and that I would be active in that process. It was all abstract, big-scheme stuff, only involving ideas and never involving me and a concrete real-life person.

But here was N. M., a real person with a pretty miserable life as it appeared to me, who seemed to enjoy having me around. And I realized that I liked that. So, when a supervisor asked me if I wanted to enroll in the next registered mental nurse training class at the hospital's school of nursing, I agreed, while secretly telling myself that I may as well do it until my perfect job came along!

Thoughts: Nursing is all about making a positive difference with individual patients. Nurses well into their careers often find themselves in roles in which they don't even glimpse actual patients for days at a time, but they realize that they can still help individual people in those roles, and that is the hook that keeps them in nursing. Florence Nightingale nursed real patients for only a relatively short period of time, and then spent fifty years organizing, educating, and writing about nursing. But without her experiences in the Crimea with those individual sick and dying soldiers, she would never have had the emotional commitment to carry on her later work.

Regretfully, I don't remember the names of some of my friends from this period, but I very clearly remember the names of many of the wonderful and weird patients whom I nursed in those first four years at this hospital.

I was one of two men in our class of about fifteen students, a lower percentage of men than in the hospital as a whole. In general, men nursing at that time constituted a very small minority, but in psychiatric hospitals in England, men were about one-third of the total number of nurses. A veteran nurse at the hospital, C. H., told me that the reason there were more men in psychiatric nursing than in general nursing dated back to the economic Great Depression of the 1930s, when working in psychiatric hospitals was one of the few career opportunities then available to men. It therefore became socially acceptable for men to enter what had been historically regarded as an exclusively female occupation and become a psychiatric nurse, a culture that carried over to subsequent generations.

When I later worked in the United States, men were still a very distinct minority in psychiatric nursing, (though still less so than in general nursing,) meaning that the culture that developed in the UK in the 1930s for some reason was not paralleled in the US.

Sketch # 2

The system at the school of nursing was that we would spend three weeks in class, and then work for the next three months on a ward appropriate to what we had learned in those classes.

After our first classroom block, I was placed on a long-term male ward, and there I first saw a man die.

Food is very important in the life of a psychiatric patient. It's one of the few pleasures they can experience, and meals were looked forward to almost as much as the cigarette breaks that were commonplace back then. On this ward, the staff got the food ready at one end of the area while the patients had to wait at the other end. When all of the food was ready, a bell would sound, and the patients would run to the food, each one determined to get his fair share of what was available.

H. K. was a man in his fifties with a diagnosis of paranoid schizophrenia, though there may also have been a touch of hypomania in the picture, and possibly also some sociopathy. He was usually buzzing about the ward, often huddling briefly with other patients, hoping to come up with secret deals with them or to scare them with whatever was on his mind at the time. With staff members, he was superficially pleasant, trying to disguise an obvious suspicion.

On this day, lunch was bangers and mash (sausages and mashed potatoes), a very popular meal, and when the bell rang, H. K. ran helter-skelter down the ward, probably hoping to finish one meal quickly and then get a second. He shoved a whole banger into his mouth, then started to cough and choke, soon turning blue. We didn't know the Heimlich maneuver or any CPR techniques at that time, so although we desperately tried to pry his jaws open and get the sausage out, we simply couldn't, and he died.

Thoughts: Meeting N. M. and then seeing a man die in front of me certainly brought home to me that I wasn't at school any more, I was in the real world. I was shocked by the death, but it wasn't new for the other staff members and the patients, and the unit emotionally sealed over surprisingly quickly.

Some anti-psychotic medications affect the gag reflex, making it difficult for some patients to reject food that they can't safely swallow, and that poses a serious risk that nurses should be aware of. Years later, when I worked at a state hospital in Massachusetts, a rash of patients died while eating hotdogs whole. The medical doctor finally ordered that all hot dogs and other meats were to be cut up into small cubes before they were given to patients. Eating little cubes of a hot dog isn't a great culinary experience, but for patients whose gag reflex isn't working properly, at least it keeps them alive.

And we should all take that annual Heimlich training seriously! Seriously!

Sketch # 3

On that same ward, P. R. was a patient. Before he had developed paranoid schizophrenia in his thirties, he had worked as a dock laborer in Southampton. Now in his fifties, he was still powerfully built, and the other patients left him pretty much alone. Staff members also tended to ask him to do things, rather than tell him as they might with the other patients. He walked stiffly and slowly, even when the meal bell rang. (He always ended up with a full plate, however.) He tended to avoid saying anything to anyone unless he had no option. He had his own chair on the ward and sat there for long periods as if deep in thought, with an occasional grimace.

During my third day on the ward, P. R. got out of his chair and slowly went to the ward bathroom and shut the door. After a few seconds, screaming came from the bathroom—truly blood-chilling screams, more frightening than anything I'd ever heard before outside of the movies.

My instinct was to go into the bathroom, as it appeared as if something truly awful was going on in there. I asked other staff members to go in with me, but they quickly told me never to go into the bathroom when P. R. was having one of these screaming sessions or he would beat me to a pulp. They said that he had frequent auditory hallucinations of boilermakers (involved in shipbuilding near the docks,) taunting and threatening him, and while he was usually able to keep control of himself, sometimes he simply couldn't. He would then go into the bathroom and scream at his reflection in the mirror for about fifteen minutes while having command hallucinations to assault any boilermaker that he met. He never destroyed any property in the bathroom, but if someone did go in, he would view him or her as one of the hated boilermakers come to challenge him and would immediately assault them.

So I listened while P. R. screamed and cursed at his invisible tormentors, threatening them with the terrible things he would do when he was finally able to confront them: "You fucking boilermakers, you just wait!...." It went on and on. That was the only patient bathroom on the ward, but not a single patient went anywhere near it. Patients and staff members alike stopped what they were doing and just listened, apparently transfixed, even though they'd heard it all many times before.

Eventually the screaming stopped, the bathroom door slowly opened, and P. R. slowly walked out to resume his position in his chair as if nothing had happened. Normal life on the ward then resumed.

Trifluperazine (trade name Stelazine) was then considered the medication of choice for the treatment of paranoid schizophrenia, and P. R. was on massive doses of it, but it obviously had limited efficacy.

Thoughts: Whenever people think about mental illness, they usually think about people having "voices" in their heads, and like many people, I had always thought of that as having a funny side to it. But hearing P. R. screaming at his voices as loud as a human being can for fifteen minutes scared me. It made me realize how terrible it must be to have auditory hallucinations, and that there was no funny side to them at all.

During my rotation on that ward, these screaming sessions happened once every three days or so. Possibly more than any other person, P. R. showed me what it meant to have a major mental illness.

There is no more dangerous time for a psychiatric nurse than to be actively working with a patient experiencing command hallucinations, as it may take very little for the patient to succumb to what the voices are telling him or her to do. Sometimes those voices tell the patient that the person standing in front of them is an enemy who must be killed, and sometimes they tell the patient that he or she should kill himself or herself. Either way, nurses should always be on highest alert for personal safety as well as patient safety.

And when a crisis breaks out and nurses don't know anything about the people involved, they shouldn't be grandiose enough to think that they know best what to do. They should listen to staff members who know the patient well and be guided by them, lest they get beaten to a pulp. When an acute situation breaks out on a unit, it can be tempting for a nurse to be a hero and do something that all of the other staff members are warning them not to do. Sometimes this may work, but more often, I have seen it result in injury to the nurse.

Sketch # 4

The remnants of an old Victorian farm were attached to the hospital, which was common with asylums of its age. These farms provided both fresh produce for the patients as well as meaningful work for many of them. In its day, the hospital farm even had a scientific spotlight on it due to a correspondence in the late 1850s between the head gardener, Henry Coe, and Charles Darwin. The data that Coe gave to Darwin regarding his experiences in growing dwarf kidney beans at the hospital farm helped Darwin develop his theory on how true plant varieties were eventually able to evolve into new varieties (4).

But when I was there, the farm was on its last legs with not a dwarf kidney bean in sight, and its role in providing patient employment was quickly being replaced by the somewhat sinister-sounding industrial therapy, involving patients making boxes and other things on the Maxwell Jones model.

But there was still a pig at the farm. One day, a small group of adolescent patients were assigned to look after the pig. For some unknown reason, they decided that day that the pig was just not pink enough for their taste, and something simply had to be done about that. They somehow were able to get hold of some neon pink paint with which they liberally daubed the pig. They then drove the creature (at times one of them riding it cowboy style) down the country lanes, yelling and whooping in triumph as they eventually entered the local village square. There the astonished local bobby stopped them, and they were returned to the hospital to proudly tell everyone the tales of their adventure for many months to come.

At our next set of school of nursing lectures, it was emphasized to us that such bizarre, spontaneous, and energetic behavior was a sure fire sign of hebephrenia, then considered a variety of teenage schizophrenia.

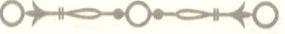

With the hospital farm having employed patients for many years, some local farmers also employed patients at harvest times, as the patients were familiar with farm work. Patients liked this, as they ended up with some money in hand as well as stomachs full of good food, and it was certainly a lot of fun for a student nurse. Several times I would go with a group of patients to pick strawberries in the fields. The farmers knew that we would eat a lot of the strawberries ourselves, but they also knew that, pretty soon, we would get sick of eating them, and then we would start filling the baskets.

Thoughts: Our diagnostic words change over time, depending upon how the causes of illnesses are viewed, but patient behaviors themselves surely don't change very much. I don't know if these particular patients went on to develop long-term psychotic disorders, but sometimes what might appear to be simply youthful hijinks may turn out to be the harbinger of something more serious developing.

Many teenagers talk about, and imagine themselves doing, bizarre things, but few actually do them, and it's worth noting for future reference when they do.

The patients' work on local farms around the hospital was an echo of a bygone age when the psychiatric hospitals and asylums in rural settings were considered legitimate parts of the local community, with a certain level of trust existing between the community and those patients able to leave the hospital. With the passing of the hospital farm, that trust between the local rural community and the hospital patients no longer exists to the same degree. That passing was probably inevitable, but seeing trust replaced by fear is regrettable.

Patients with a schizophrenic illness have great difficulty in forming any positive emotional attachment to other people. They are so guarded in their emotions that no relationship can truly flourish, and they often go through life friendless.

But there seems to be in everyone a biological need to nurture or have some other sort of relationship with another living thing, even if that's not a human being. So patients with schizophrenia sometimes greatly enjoy growing flowers and vegetables. For them it is an acceptable and nonthreatening relationship.

Years later I visited a very interesting garden and greenhouse in a state hospital in Massachusetts. Patients were growing and selling exotic plants. And when I worked at another hospital, in Ohio, the occupational therapy department organized a successful vegetable garden tended by patients, a garden that sadly had to be abandoned when the old buildings were razed and the hospital was rebuilt specifically as a forensic psychiatric hospital.

It's the same with animals. When I worked at a hospital in Boston, Massachusetts, an old nurse told us about a cat who had lived on the unit years before—a cat that was fussed over by all of the patients, but perhaps particularly so by the schizophrenic patients. These patients would be almost phobic regarding physical contact with other humans, but petting a cat posed no emotional dangers to them and seemed to satisfy that primal human need to have a relationship of some sort.

Sketch # 5

In the early 1970s, the cast of the television show, *Monty Python's Flying Circus*, was doing a tour of Britain and were coming to the Odeon, a theatre in Southampton. I had been a big fan of Monty Python since my college days and was desperate to go. Of course, by Murphy's Law, my work schedule had me working at the hospital that evening. I therefore proposed to the treatment team of the ward I was working on at the time to let me take some patients to the show, providing they were considered safe to go and wanted to go.

So, I ended up taking four patients along with me. We laughed at the familiar skits involving The Ministry of Funny Walks and The Dead Parrot and so forth. But then a skit came on which involved someone being cut into thin slices—sort of like slicing a tomato for a hamburger. In the middle of that, one of the patients suddenly started screaming and ran out of the theater. I went out after him, eventually catching up with him in the street, and tried to calm him down. After a while, he said that he had a constant thought (delusion) that he had never told anyone about—that of being killed one day in an exactly similar manner as portrayed in the skit. He had become frightened that they were going to call him up onto the stage and kill him there, so he had run out. After some time, we were able to go back to the show where I was very relieved to see the other patients still sitting there, and for their part I think that they were also relieved to see both of us.

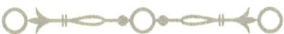

In that era, long-stay patients were almost routinely allowed to go off the hospital grounds for a pass when an opportunity presented itself, as most of them were no longer considered as safety risks; there was just no places to discharge them to. All that was needed was someone willing to go with them. In this current era, the outlook is quite different, with the emphasis being that, if a patient is able to go on a pass, he or she is able to be discharged.

I was a big soccer fan and would often take a patient (usually a long-stay patient) with me when I was going to a game, particularly a Portsmouth game, as the hospital was on the way from my apartment to their stadium. Patients who had been hospitalized for years were clearly a little disorientated when we were out of the hospital engaged in what would be normal activities for everyone else, and stuck close to me rather than trying to escape. I think that they enjoyed the games, even if they were often anxious about what was generally going on around them, and when we returned to the hospital, they expressed a mixture of regret and relief.

Thoughts: If we're lucky, patients will tell us about some of their most fearful delusions. But even then, what they will tell us is probably only the tip of their iceberg; most of it they will keep to themselves. Psychiatric nurses must expect the unexpected because they rarely fully know their patients.

I have seen truly "institutionalized" patients, who had been hospitalized for decades, discharged into the community, usually under the pressure of the cost of keeping them in hospital, but also sometimes because treatment teams idealistically believed that a successful discharge was possible. My experience has been that this most often fails, as the patients simply cannot cope with the constant and unfamiliar anxieties of what is everyday life to the rest of us. It then seems a kindness to let them live out their lives in hospital (see Sketch #78). But money, in the end, is, of course, the deciding factor in many health care issues. For instance, in the United States, poorer rural counties may be faced with spending millions of dollars on the care of one chronic, severely mentally ill resident of their county—money that they simply can't afford. They then must try to discharge the patient whenever an opportunity arises, even if they know that the patient will very likely be back in the hospital a few weeks later, as the tax-payer money thus saved is important for their budget.

Sketch # 6

The registered mental nurse training was three years long and qualified graduates to work as staff nurses only in a psychiatric setting. During that time, we had a three-month rotation in a general hospital so that we would be able to take care of the medical and surgical needs of our psychiatric patients.

During my rotation in a Southampton general hospital, we were being given our assignments one morning by the ward sister (charge nurse) at the start of the shift. One of my assignments was to give Mr. J. in room forty-eight an enema. However, when I went to Mr. J.'s room, he was quite dead; in fact, he was in rigor mortis. My thinking went along the lines of: *Well, they must know that he's dead after this length of time, so clearing out his bowels must be a part of the postmortem process that I just don't know about.*

So I wrestled Mr. J. onto his side and gave him his enema, with some actual positive results! I then asked one of the staff nurses what I should do next regarding their postmortem protocol. When she realized what I had done, she burst out laughing and hurried off to tell the other nurses what the foolish psychiatric nursing student had just done. I was embarrassed about it, of course, and was razzed about it for some time by my classmates. But other than their initial reaction, the incident was rarely mentioned again by the general hospital nurses, as everyone there knew that some staff nurse had gone home without realizing that one of her patients had been dead for several hours, and people were keen for that to be left unspoken.

It was during this rotation that I started to call patients by their titles—Mr. Smith and Mrs. Jones—rather than only by their first names, which is what staff traditionally do in psychiatric nursing. If patients asked me to call them by their first names, then I happily did so, but otherwise I used their titles. It just seemed more respectful to me. It has been my experience that adult patients (including those in their late teens) prefer to be called by their title rather than their first name. There's a basic social element of politeness and respect involved here, and we shouldn't simply assume that we automatically have the right to call patients by their first name.

Thought: Nurses must not automatically accept that people with more authority than them must automatically be up to date with everything that's happening on their unit. Nurses must always check with their supervisor if something just seems weird to them!

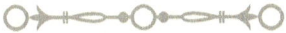

Sketch # 7

After a while, I was assigned a rotation on the night shift at the hospital, on a long-stay male ward. The regular night nurse was a man in his forties, a night-shift lifer, cheerful and talkative, which I appreciated, as it helped keep me awake.

Mr. C. was a patient in his late fifties, diagnosed with Huntington's disease and dementia. Seemingly every part of his body would be writhing and jerking, so our hearts were in our mouths every time he got up to walk, as it appeared inevitable that he would fall down. Yet he never did.

During the night, Mr. C. would sometimes get up and try to convince various staff members to give him something extra to eat. But this very rarely worked, as the staff figured that, if they did it for him, soon many patients would be up requesting the same. Patients do have an uncanny knack of picking up on that sort of thing very quickly.

One night, Mr. C. was particularly persistent in asking for food, and he was starting to become quite agitated. After saying no several times, the nurse suddenly punched him hard in the stomach and yelled at him to get back to bed. Which he did.

The nurse then went on to explain to me that this was the only way to handle this patient when he became agitated like that, as eventually he would become so loud that he would wake up all of the other patients. It was clear that what had just happened had happened many times before, though I was the only witness to this assault.

I was shocked by what I'd seen but was also quite uncertain regarding what I should do about it. I knew that the assault should be reported and the nurse should properly be fired. At the same time, I anxiously wondered what would happen to me at the hospital once it was known by all of the other staff that I had got an established and popular nurse fired.

I was also actively involved in the union at the hospital, the Confederation of Health Services Employees, and it didn't seem that a union official should be initiating a process that might end up with a fellow union member being fired.

So I did nothing.

Thought: Nurses should always do what they know is the right thing because, if they don't, they'll think about it on and off for the rest of their lives, wishing they had done the right thing.

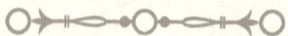

At this time in Britain, there was developing competition between various organizations over recruitment of registered nurses (RNs). The Royal College of Nursing was the traditional organization representing professional nursing, and most RNs automatically joined it even though it was widely regarded as being a "snobby" organization.

But it was then being challenged by health care unions which viewed themselves as representing the interests of the still relatively new National Health Service and wanted to recruit everyone who worked in the NHS in order to ensure the survival of what was essentially a social experiment, not just nurses.

So, unions like the Confederation of Health Service Employees represented groups such as housekeepers, cooks, plant and operations workers, and unlicensed nursing staff, but also any professional staff members who might choose to join them, such as RNs or the occasional medical doctor.

At the time, it made sense to me that what was good for the NHS was automatically good for nurses, so joining a union that represented more than just nurses was the right thing to do. However, over the years my experience was that these unions ended up subordinating the professional interests of nurses to their bigger union goals to the extent that, in practice, professional nursing standards ended up being eroded. I knew some nurses who behaved quite unprofessionally and who knew that they were behaving unprofessionally, but were not unduly concerned, confidently believing that the union would "get them off."

Even in unions that represented only nurses or nurses and other health professions, no matter what might be stated about professionalism in the literature, the actual leaders of the union at the local level and beyond tended to be people who were personally more motivated in promoting the broader goals of the trade union movement than to advancing the professionalism of nursing.

Sketch # 8

I was assigned to the admission ward at the hospital during my second year of training. One day I was astonished to see a patient walk onto the ward who looked more like I imagined Robinson Crusoe would look like than anyone I expected to see in the 1970s. He wore old shoes without laces, no socks, dirty trousers cut off at the knees, and was bare chested. He had a long, straggly beard and hair, with feathers, twigs, and other odd items stuck in them with apparently some thought. He was very cheerful, very talkative, and just bursting at the seams with energy.

Mr. T. was my first introduction to what was then called manic depressive illness, now known as bipolar disorder, in an untreated manic state.

He was in his early thirties and had been in the hospital once several years before but had apparently received no psychiatric care for his illness for a long time.

At that time lithium and haloperidol (trade name Haldol) were the medications of choice for mania, and while Mr. T. was happy enough to take them, his mania was at such a pitch that there was little immediate response to them. Meanwhile, his thoughts were spinning around in his head so fast that he would forget to do the basics of life, such as eating and drinking. So one of the assignments given to us student nurses was to trot behind him as he strode about the ward, carrying some water and a small snack with us, trying to get him to get him to take something so that he didn't end up being in a medical crisis due to dehydration.

But his energy level tired us all out, and until the medications finally kicked in, a way had to be found to let him work off some of that energy. The treatment team came up with the seemingly odd idea of giving him a spade letting him just dig away with no real aim in mind. But it worked wonderfully!

So for several days, after breakfast, Mr. T. would be given a spade. Off he would march to the hospital farm a couple of hundred yards away. There he was shown some vacant plots of land, and he would just start digging away. Every half hour he would be asked to stop and would be given something to eat and drink, and then he'd be back to it, just digging and digging. He never tried to escape and always came back to the unit in the late afternoon.

Eventually the medications started to slow Mr. T. down. He no longer needed to go out digging on the farm and could stay on the unit. After six weeks, he was discharged as stable.

Thought: We rarely see a completely untreated manic patient admitted these days, as somewhere along the line they've had some form of treatment, even if it's just recent intramuscular medications in an emergency room. Seeing this patient in such a state made me realize how very difficult it must have been to care for such patients in the old asylum days before psychiatric medications were developed. And later on, I was to learn that mania with euphoric mood is a lot more enjoyable and less problematic to care for than mania with dysphoric mood!

Sketch # 9

One day at the admission unit, we received a call from Mr. P., who simply said, "She's done it again. I think that you need to come out here." The nurse didn't ask for any more details; she just replied that we'd be there as soon as we could.

As I rode out with the nurse who assessed admission referrals, she explained the situation to me. The caller was the husband of a patient in her early sixties who was diagnosed with Capgras syndrome. This was a pretty rare diagnosis. Patients were otherwise quite functional, but every now and then they became consumed by the delusion that someone important in their lives (usually a close family member) was an identical-looking impostor, not the real person.

In this case, about every two years or so, Mrs. P. began to become convinced that her husband of nearly forty years was an impostor, and then he had to leave the house for his own safety as she usually threatened to attack him with a kitchen knife if he didn't leave.

When we got to the house, Mr. P. was sitting resignedly on a box on the front lawn. Some of his clothes and belongings were scattered about where his wife had thrown them out. Mrs. P. was peeping out from behind the curtains of the front room.

"It's worse than usual this time," Mr. P. told us. "I suppose she hasn't been talking her pills, though I thought she had."

The nurse knew Mrs. P. well and eventually persuaded her to open the door and then to come back with us to the hospital. As we drove away, Mr. P. was starting to collect his clothes from the lawn and take them inside.

Mrs. P. was given her antipsychotic medications at the hospital and was discharged after about four weeks. I was told that she fondly embraced her husband when she was taken home.

Thoughts: This was a particularly interesting case to me because, although it was a serious mental illness, the patient could be reasonably functional for most of her life, only periodically becoming disabled by a single, encapsulated, powerful delusion. Usually delusions end up including so many areas of patients' lives that they become unable to conduct their lives in any well-functioning manner. But this particular disorder has just the one focus—that a close associate is an impostor. Capgras syndrome is now incorporated into the larger diagnosis of paranoid schizophrenia.

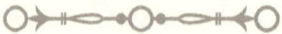

As I look back on it, I realize that there was a generally relaxed approach to early 1970s psychiatry England that, for risk management purposes, could never be replicated now. Now, a nurse would never bring an acutely ill patient for admission to the hospital in her own car, and with no police involvement. Such a potentially dangerous incident just wouldn't happen now. But whatever everyone accepts as being the way in which things are done ends up being the best way of doing them, and in the 1970s this was a perfectly effective process.

Sketch # 10

Another patient who came to the admission ward was Ms. P. She was in her early twenties and had been diagnosed with schizoaffective disorder. Young as she was, she was already well known to the ward staff members, having been admitted several times already, sometimes for suicidal ideation. This time around, she was angry, agitated, and probably having auditory hallucinations, though she denied it. She stomped around the ward, glowering at staff members and ignoring other patients.

She was also blonde, pretty, and my age.

After a while I began to find myself thinking about her more and more, even when I was at home and away from work. Eventually I asked her if I could see her after she had been discharged from the hospital. It was a mixture of sexual attraction and grandiose thinking on my part that I personally could help stabilize her illness and halt her continued deterioration, should I have a relationship with her.

After I asked her, she stared at me for a while then contemptuously turned and stalked away, saying nothing. A few days later, she walked up to me on the ward and slapped my face. None of the other staff members could figure out why on earth she had done it, but I knew.

Thoughts: Sexual and other boundary violations between psychiatric nurses and patients are serious dangers that come with the job yet are rarely satisfactorily addressed by schools of nursing. When this incident occurred, we had never heard anything about it in class, so when I started often thinking about Ms. P., no alarms started going off in my head.

At best, boundary violations with regular psychiatric patients makes their effective treatment almost impossible. And at worst, such violations with forensic psychiatric patients who may be actively seeking to exploit unprofessional behavior and vulnerabilities on the part of staff may produce disastrous results.

This is something that schools of nursing should be addressing with students in their first few months of training. Student nurses must be told that, as one of the pitfalls of the job, they shouldn't keep an attraction a secret; rather, they should talk openly about it with their supervisors. Then it can be worked out as a legitimate clinical issue before it becomes a legal issue that may end up ending nursing careers.

Even for nurses who want a "planned" boundary crossing, such as when I took patients to soccer games, the key is to talk to their supervisors about it, and to make sure that the patients' treatment teams know about and approve the activity. I exchanged Christmas cards for forty years with two patients I first knew at this hospital, but I first made sure that everyone knew when I started doing it.

In classical psycho-analysis, my feelings toward this patient would have been described as being counter transference. Meaning that, due to her mental illness, the patient started to develop a distorted view and have distorted unconscious feelings about me (that is transference), and then I unconsciously developed my feelings as a response to hers (counter transference.) In this theory, the problem therefore always starts with the patient, with the health professional simply reacting to that problem. This theory may conveniently provide cover for a professional person acting badly, but it didn't apply to the above scenario, or to many others that I have seen.

In this case, Ms. P. was simply being Ms. P.; the feelings that I started to develop toward her were entirely my affair and my responsibility.

Sketch # 11

Mr. K. was in his early thirties, and this was his fourth admission to the hospital. His diagnosis was manic depressive (bipolar) disorder, and this time he was hypomanic (his symptoms were the same but less severe than they would be if he were manic). This was most clearly evidenced by his psychotic thinking rather than any hyperactivity, although he was constantly restless.

He was an electrician by trade and had fixed up one of the rooms in his house with additional electrical outlets. He would then turn on all of the switches and stand in the middle of the room with his hands in the air, imagining himself to be then absorbing power from the outlets as if he were a super hero.

He was also paranoid about his work colleagues, thinking they conspired against him. And he was paranoid about the doctors at the hospital, believing that they were misdiagnosing him and giving him the wrong medications. He once filed a law suit against the hospital on this issue, a very rare occurrence in England at that time.

In the past, he had been suicidal when in his depressive phase, and there was some evidence that he and his mother had once had a suicide pact that his mother had carried out, but he had not. He had been married but was now divorced.

In a hypomanic phase, he had been able to obtain UK, US, and Irish passports for himself.

His admission was uneventful, although he relentlessly struggled over which medications he should take, and what their dosages should be. As with many bipolar patients, he liked being slightly manic, feeling much better in that state than when he was depressed or when his mood was euthymic ("normal"). He therefore deliberately and carefully tried to adjust the dosage of his medication so that he didn't become ill enough to require hospitalization, yet was manic enough to feel powerful and exhilarated.

I've known a number of patients who have tried to pull this delicate trick off, but he was the only one I knew who actually did it. He was successfully able to keep himself stable enough to work for many years in a manufacturing plant as an electrician without requiring hospitalization, yet manic enough to be able to work a lot of overtime and earn a lot of money.

Thought: Although he was grandiose and paranoid when hypomanic, Mr. K. was actually a popular patient with his peers and with staff members. People simply liked him, and he liked people. I learned that this ability to connect emotionally with other people is a good way of diagnostically distinguishing a mood-disordered patient from a purely schizophrenic patient, when both present with the same psychotic symptoms. People with schizophrenia are rarely able to make positive, meaningful, emotional connections with their fellow humans, while mood-disordered patients usually are.

Sketch # 12

Once a week the treatment team on the admission ward would meet during rounds to review the progress of each patient. Everyone would gradually gather a few minutes before the assigned time, but nothing really happened until the consultant (the psychiatrist in charge of the ward) came in. When he sat down, the sister would then ceremonially bring in a tray with a pot of hot tea, a cup and saucer, milk, and sugar, and place it on a table beside him. Rounds could then begin.

One week the consultant shocked us all by suddenly starting to loudly yell at sister in front of everyone gathered there. It turned out that the cause for this was that, while sister had put the milk and sugar in the tea for him, she had neglected to stir it. The consultant apparently felt that this was not a duty to be performed by a physician and must have assumed that his response would be approved of by everyone else in the room as being perfectly justified, rather than our being appalled by his arrogant and boorish behavior.

On the other hand, another consultant, Dr. S. B., presented nurses with the best side of a psychiatrist. He had worked at the hospital for many years and knew that many things that we might wish for in our work were simply unlikely to happen in a National Health Service psychiatric hospital. Patiently, thoughtfully, and good-humoredly he went about plying his trade every day. He was about sixty years old and apparently had no desire to fill any other role than being a unit psychiatrist. I enjoyed watching him at work, and he played a large part in helping me eventually realize that, in psychiatric nursing, I might actually already have found my perfect job.

Thought: There are good and bad people in every group. We should all try to focus on the good ones and learn what we can from them while we are with them.

This hospital closed in 1996.

CHAPTER 2

A Midlands, UK, Hospital

Sketch # 13

After three years, I graduated as a Registered Mental Nurse. I never thought at all about the wording of that title until I started working in the United States. When I told people there that I was a registered mental nurse, they would often start laughing, interpreting that noble title along the lines of someone being, for instance, a registered sex offender. The idea of having a special governmental register for "mental" nurses was indeed funny, and I soon stopped telling people about my RMN status!

I started working as a staff nurse at the Hampshire hospital, but after six months, although I had many wonderful experiences there, I got an itch to see something different. The trend in psychiatry at that time, in an effort to reduce the stigma of mental illness, was to move away from treating patients in large hospitals and treat them, instead, in small units in general hospitals.

So, in 1975, I went to work at the psychiatric unit at a hospital in the Midlands. I had lived in my own apartment when I was in Hampshire, but for convenience and to save money, I lived at the hospitals' nurses' home while I was there. The nurses' home was divided into men's and women's sections, but I was assigned an apartment with two women nurses, a daring administrative move at that time.

The psychiatric unit where I worked was a small one of fifteen beds, run as a treatment and teaching tool for the medical students and residents at a Midlands university. It was the child of perhaps the smartest person I ever knew, Dr. T. W., later Sir T.

"The Prof," as the staff all referred to him, held weekly rounds to review the patients on the unit, and the conference room was always crammed at that time, with everyone fascinated to see The Prof in action interviewing and diagnosing patients. He was a big man. Sitting comfortably in his chair, he reminded me of Sidney Greenstreet in the old movie *The Maltese Falcon*.

When interviewing patients, he could zero in to the crux of their illnesses as if by instinct, which none of us could ever replicate no matter how hard we tried. He knew exactly when to push his questions and when to back off. He was idiosyncratic in his use of alcohol with some psychiatric disorders; he ordered a schooner (a large glass) of sherry before meals for his anorexic patients in the belief that this stimulated the appetite, and a bottle of Guinness (Irish stout) before bedtime for the geriatric patients who had difficulty sleeping. I didn't really see the sherry as having much positive effect, but the older patients loved the Guinness, and they slept pretty soundly after drinking it.

One week in rounds, he surprised us all by not interviewing a particular patient at all. He simply listened to her history and behaviors as presented by the resident and nursing staff, and then, when she came into the rounds room, he made only a single declaration to her.

This patient had been admitted to the unit from the hospital's emergency room with a provisional diagnosis of what was then called Munchausen's syndrome, now known as factitious disorder. She was in her mid-thirties and had gone to the emergency room complaining of chest pain. Initial tests came up as negative, so she was probably going to be discharged unless something else turned up. Then, as a nurse was pulling back the curtain from the patient's bed, she noticed the patient surreptitiously taking some pills from a bottle. The patient then tried to hide the bottle, but after a brief tussle, the nurse was able to get it.

The pills turned out to be potassium. The patient was trying to artificially induce dangerous cardiac arrhythmias in herself so that she would be admitted to the hospital. At that point, she was gastrically lavaged (her stomached was pumped) and then sent to the psychiatric unit.

When she came into rounds, The Prof simply looked at her intensely for a while then said, "Madam, I know what troubles you. I can cure you. But you must stay. Will you stay? Let me know by tomorrow." She was then ushered out of the room.

We were all shocked, as we had expected a penetrating interview to help us gain some insight into this baffling behavior. The Prof then explained, "People who live this way have absolutely no interest in living any other way. Being involved in constant medical dramas is what they crave above anything else. She will be gone by tomorrow. Would anyone like to have a small wager with me on this?"

There was a long silence as he waited to see if anyone would take up his challenge. I eventually did. I just couldn't understand why a person living such a wretched life would not jump at the chance of possibly having that life transformed. I believed at that time that all patients must know that they had an illness and that they surely all wanted to be cured. So I bet The Prof one pound that she would stay.

The Prof was wrong only in that she didn't even wait until the next day; she signed herself out within an hour.

Thoughts: My thinking that all patients know that they are ill and want to be cured was the hopeful thinking of a nurse still new to the field, but regrettably it is far from being true. Indeed, one of the confounding issues in psychiatry is patients with particularly psychotic disorders who discontinue their medications even though every logic would tell them that it will be only a matter of time before they will end up back in hospital or even jail. They mainly discontinue their medications not because of side effects or some other reason they might have, but largely because, in their hearts, they simply do not believe that they have a mental illness and therefore need no treatment.

At that time, every emergency room sister (charge nurse) had a "little black book" containing the names of Munchausen patients with whom they had been involved in the past, so they could be forewarned should the patient appear again for treatment. The contents of these books were also known to be shared between emergency rooms in the same general locality. Ethically and legally such documents should not exist, of course, but I wonder if some version of them still do.

As an additional note, we should never bet against a smart man who's talking about his area of expertise!

Sketch # 14

Mr. F. was a man in his late sixties, recently widowed, and admitted with a diagnosis of psychotic depression. He was frail and had a poor appetite and a poor sleep pattern. He always looked preoccupied and avoided talking to staff members if he could. He denied having suicidal intentions.

A few days later when I came on duty one morning, the night staff reported that Mr. F. had died that night. The night shift consisted of a practical nurse and a nursing assistant. It was fashionable in that era to have doors of psychiatric units open, the rationale being that this helped to combat the culture of treating patients as dangerous lunatics who needed to be locked up.

This unit's entrance doors had therefore also been open, though it was the duty of staff members to constantly observe the door to make sure that no patient actually walked out.

What the night staff told us was that Mr. F. had somehow gone down the corridor leading to the entrance doors and then through the doors without their noticing it. They said that they had soon noticed that he was not on the unit, and after quickly searching the unit unsuccessfully, they had gone off the unit to look for him.

They found him lying dead just outside the unit doors; his skull was broken in several places. They told the hospital night supervisor that he must have simply tripped and cracked his head. That was accepted as being apparently most likely what happened, so it was not treated as a police matter.

However, later that day, the picture changed dramatically. The unit was on the fifth floor of the hospital, and just outside of the entrance doors was a stairwell leading to the lower floors. An alert young resident walking up those stairs that morning noticed something on one of the steps, and he couldn't figure out what it was. When he took a closer look, he soon realized that what he was looking at was some skull fragments and brain tissue.

The police were then alerted and went out to the houses of the two night-shift staff members to interview them.

The story that then emerged was this: Mr. F. had indeed quietly left the unit when the night staff had not been watching. He had then most likely climbed onto the safety railings on the fifth floor above the stairwell and then, in a successful suicide attempt, jumped head first onto the steps leading to the fourth floor.

When the night staff realized that he was not on the unit, they searched the area outside and found him dead on the stairs. Panicked that they would be fired for not seeing him leave the unit to kill himself, they thought up a plan to carry the body back up the stairs and place it outside the unit doors, and then claim that he had tripped when leaving the unit. They thought that they had cleaned the stairs of all of the blood and tissue left after the fall but had not noticed that one piece.

After an investigation, the staff members were fired, but legal charges were not filed.

Thoughts: If a patient presents theoretically as a suicide risk, nurses must assume that he or she is, no matter what he or she may say to the contrary.

Regarding the staff, what they did was legally and professionally unacceptable, yet I couldn't help feeling sorry for them in some ways. They were both women in their early sixties who needed to earn money. When they discovered Mr. F.'s body, they believed that they would be fired and never get a job in nursing again. They panicked, and in their panic, did a very foolish thing. As is usually said regarding politics, the cover-up ends up being worse for the participants than what they were covering up in the first place.

If the unit door had been locked, this suicide would most likely have been avoided, but in that era of psychiatry, even an acute admission unit had to have an open unit or it did not meet the theoretical requirements of a therapeutic milieu. Patient safety was, in reality, a secondary consideration, and remained so until the subsequent era of biological psychiatry, when unit doors at last were locked again.

Sketch # 15

One day, a patient in his mid-fifties was admitted to the unit, a transfer from a medical-surgical unit at the hospital. He had initially been admitted to that unit with complaints of abdominal pain, but an initial workup there found no physical reason for this pain, so he had then been transferred to the psychiatric unit.

The psychodynamic theory behind this was that some people are unable to show their emotional pain openly for personal or cultural reasons, and therefore show the pain in a physical way. Sometimes depressed patients present as being psychosomatic with unexplained aches and pains all over, and this patient's treatment team felt that his pain must be of a similar psychic origin.

On the psychiatric unit, the patient would have periods of writhing about on the floor clutching his abdomen and calling out for help. The unit psychologist formulated a treatment plan for him based on not rewarding his expression of pain physically but rewarding his discussing emotions that might be painful to him.

What happened, therefore, was that, when the patient was writhing about on the floor, groaning and calling for help, we totally ignored him, including stepping over him if he was lying in one of the unit corridors. This was quite unnerving to us, but we believed it was the right thing to do as we believed the theory that the pain that was causing him to act in this way was emotional rather than physical.

Nothing changed with his behavior, though, and his claims of violent spasms of pain even appeared to become worse. Eventually, a new resident on the unit got permission to have a laparotomy done just to make doubly sure that there was no physical cause for the pain. (A laparotomy is a surgical investigation of the abdominal cavity.)

After the laparotomy, we were told that the patient was riddled with cancer so advanced that any treatment would be useless. He was therefore just sewn up again and transferred back to a medical-surgical unit, where he died three weeks later.

Thought: There was plenty of shame and guilt to pass around over this terrible case, and we psychiatric unit staff members felt our share very keenly. As nurses supposedly dedicated to meeting the needs of our patients, we had been deliberately ignoring the pleas of a dying man who was in extreme pain—all because of a psychiatric theory. Up to that time, I had been excited the by psychodynamic model of behavior generally prevalent at that time, but after this case, I began to lose some confidence that we in psychiatry actually knew what we were talking about.

Two years later, I experienced a similar sort of case in a Boston, Massachusetts, hospital's outpatient clinic. There a patient started falling down and asking for staff members to help him get up. An initial physical workup showed no apparent cause for this, so staff were told that, when he had these falls and couldn't get up, he was acting out some hidden emotional conflicts. Once we had uncovered these psychic conflicts, the falling would stop, so the theory went. Staff members therefore ignored him when he fell and begged for help to get back up, again stepping over him if necessary. But the falling went on, so eventually a second physical work up was ordered. This revealed that the patient had developed multiple sclerosis.

So, nurses must be very careful when colleagues declare that a patient's behavior is simply attention seeking. It may be attention seeking, but it may also be something else entirely.

Sketch # 16

On the other hand, there are certainly patient behaviors that really are attention seeking, and are best managed as such.

Ms. A. was eighteen years old with an established diagnosis of temporal lobe epilepsy and a mild intellectual disability (5). Her seizures had been well controlled on the anti-seizure medication carbamazepine (trade name Tegretol) for several years, but her parents had recently reported an inexplicable surge in seizure activity. She had therefore been admitted to a medical unit at the hospital, and when their tests suggested no change in her epileptic status, she was transferred to the psychiatric unit for evaluation of potential psychogenic seizures.

On the unit, she showed two apparently distinct types of epileptic seizures. About once a week, she had the classical tonic-clonic seizure with urinary incontinence and a slow, confused recovery.

The other seizure type occurred about six times a day, always taking place in front of other people in the main unit corridor. It was noted that these often followed her participation in occupational therapy activities involving games or quizzes. During these, she would fall gracefully to the floor and thrash randomly around, loudly moaning and shouting. After a minute or two, she would stop, get up in apparently clear consciousness, and ask staff members what had happened to her.

These latter seizures were diagnosed as being "hysterical" in nature, and staff members were instructed to ignore them so as not to give her any positive reinforcement to have them. We also told her that she need not attend the occupational therapy sessions in the hope that this would eliminate the embarrassment and self-consciousness that she may have experienced during activities in which she could not perform as well as other patients.

Initially the seizures became more frequent, the thrashing about more violent, the yelling louder, and the duration of the episodes longer (one lasted nearly an hour). However, after about a week, they were occurring at the rate of one a day, and after another week, had stopped altogether.

Her carbamazepine dosage was increased, resulting in her then having no seizures at all, and she was discharged.

Thought: Occasionally patients with genuine epilepsy do have hysterical seizures in addition to the real ones; this often is associated with an intellectual disability. Patients appear to be unable to express anger, frustration, and similar emotions in the usual verbal ways, and end up acting out these feelings behaviorally, using their experience of having genuine seizures as the template for these behaviors.

For the psychiatric nurse, it's usually fairly easy to spot the difference between the two types of seizure. But as the previous sketch shows, all of the appropriate tests should be done, and everyone on the treatment team should fully agree before ignoring a patient's behavior as a deliberate treatment strategy. And even then, it should always be remembered that the evaluation might be faulty, particularly if the patient behavior does not improve in response to being ignored.

A veteran nurse once told me never to stand bending over a patient who was having a seizure. His reasoning was that, when such patients recover consciousness they are very confused and are unable to understand why they are lying on the ground. If they then see someone standing over them, they may well assume that this person has assaulted them—that's why they are on the ground—and they may then assault whoever is standing over them in return. So I have always been careful not to get within arm's length of a patient recovering from a seizure.

Sketch # 17

Alcoholic patients were sometimes admitted to the unit for an initial detoxification, after which they would be placed on a disulfiram (trade name Antabuse) regime. People who drink alcohol while taking disulfiram feel physically very ill. It's a bit like having the worst hangover ever. The idea, of course, is that this provides the incentive not to drink.

The psychologist taught us to "reinforce" to the patient the dire consequences of drinking while taking this medication in order to make them fearful of doing so and thus remain sober. So once a day in the days leading up to the patient's discharge, and more frequently in the two days before discharge, three or four staff members would take the patient into a room and have him or her sit in a chair, while staff members also sat down. We would then take turns telling the patient of the awful symptoms that he would experience should he take alcohol while on disulfiram: "Don't do it! You'll have a terrible headache." "You'll be sick all over the place." "You'll feel like you're dying, and you *will* die if you go into circulatory collapse." And so it went.

We were taught to bark this out aggressively to the patient, bordering on yelling, as if it was an FBI interrogation session of the sort that you see on TV, in order to emphasize the point to the patient. Drinking alcohol while also taking disulfiram may well be medically dangerous, but the primary theory behind these sessions was to instill an active degree of fear in patients of doing both, and therefore help keep them sober.

The obvious flaw in the treatment is that alcoholics who want to drink again simply stop taking the drug. Looking back on it, our sessions may have simply convinced them that discontinuing the disulfiram was the safest route to take. Other alcoholics have since told me that they did drink while also taking disulfiram, but found that the medical effects were much milder than they anticipated, so they continued drinking.

Thought: Even in well-meaning endeavors, patients can eventually figure out that care givers appear to be exaggerating their point. The backlash then is that the whole project is dismissed—baby and bathwater alike.

Sketch # 18

A young man in his early twenties was admitted with a provisional diagnosis of schizophrenia, not otherwise specified. He was isolated on the unit, saying little to anyone, but showing no obvious signs or symptoms of psychosis.

After being on the unit a day or two, he appeared to become preoccupied with his right hand, staring at it silently for literally hours at a time. Whenever a staff member would ask about this, he would stare at them as if he didn't understand the question and make no reply.

When The Prof was in one day, we told him about this and asked him what he thought was going on with the patient. His reply was, "It's the hand that he masturbates with. He's probably wondering whether or not he should cut it off. But he won't."

After about three weeks, as the medications started to take effect, the patient started to slowly lose interest in his hand and was then discharged.

Years later, I knew a patient with schizophrenia who had castrated himself. He said that he felt limited pain while doing it—mainly numbness—a truly extraordinary example of mind over matter. If one day we can figure out the biochemical processes that occurs during an active psychosis that makes a person virtually immune to extreme pain, what an advance we could then make in many areas of life!

Thought: Control is a big issue in everyone's life, but perhaps particularly so in people with schizophrenia, who may view their normal urges and their effects as direct threats to their own self-control. Sexual urges may seem frightening and overwhelming to them, and occasionally their answer to that is to mutilate themselves in order to eliminate this threat to their control.

When Emil Kraepelin popularized the term "dementia praecox" in the 1890s for what we now call schizophrenia, he believed that the organic changes in the patient's brain had probably been caused by being flooded by sex hormones when the patient was in adolescence. Perhaps observing patients such as this young man gave him that idea.

Sketch # 19

A man in his early forties was admitted to the unit complaining that he was having thoughts of homosexual activity with other men. These thoughts greatly distressed him, and he wanted us to stop them from happening.

The psychologist therefore drew up a "graduated desensitization program" to achieve the patient's stated goal. This consisted of having him lie down in a quiet, darkened room with a male nurse sitting a few yards away who would soothingly tell the patient that he was slowly becoming completely relaxed. The patient was to say nothing but would signal his sense of relaxation to the staff member by raising a single finger. He was then to talk about his sexual thoughts while the staff member soothingly reassured him that nothing sexual would actually happen as a result of these thoughts.

These sessions were done twice daily for about a week but were discontinued when the patient stated that he was actually becoming more sexually aroused by the sessions themselves than by his own thoughts.

Thought: Care givers should never be grandiose enough to think that they have theories powerful enough to change what can't be changed.

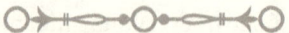

When I later worked at a south London hospital, I did see a graduated desensitization program work well. This involved a woman in her late fifties who had developed agoraphobia following the death of her parents and the emigration of her only child to Australia. She first became anxious when she left her apartment to go shopping, and this developed to panic when she needed to catch a bus and had to wait for a few minutes. She was started on diazepam (trade name Valium) as an outpatient with little success and was eventually admitted to the inpatient unit. She remained on diazepam but also started a program involving staff members accompanying her on gradually longer and longer walks outside of the hospital. After six weeks, she was able to walk from the hospital to her apartment by herself and was then discharged (6).

Sketch # 20

A man in his late sixties was admitted with a provisional diagnosis of dementia, but who needed full psychiatric and physical workups.

From the first day, every few hours he would have periods lasting for about five minutes during which time he would agitatedly walk up and down the main corridor yelling "Ahhhhhhhh … ahhhhhhh … ahhhhhhh." All attempts by staff members to get him to calm down simply resulted in him yelling louder and longer.

We were soon telling the charge nurse, "He doesn't belong here. This is a psychiatric unit not a nursing home!" They implored him to get the patient discharged. When The Prof came on the unit, we all gathered round him to tell him how agitated the new patient was making the other patients, and we explained why we thought he should therefore be quickly discharged.

The Prof knew that, when we said that a patient was agitating the other patients, what we really meant was that he or she was agitating us! He asked us if we thought that it would be right to discharge a patient while we were still just guessing what was going on with him, and we sheepishly agreed that it wouldn't. He said that the yelling would probably lessen as the patient became familiar with the unit, and he promised to look at the patient's medication regime to see if something could be added that would help calm him down.

Over the next three weeks, the patient had all of the tests and assessments needed to make a definitive diagnosis, and his yelling did abate quite a bit. But we could never entirely shed our underlying anger about him being on the unit, an anger that remained until he was transferred to a nursing home.

Thoughts: On a psychiatric unit, it's not uncommon for staff members to say amongst themselves and to the manager: "Wouldn't the unit be great if only patient X wasn't here?" (Not by coincidence, patient X often has a mental disability or dementia, which psychiatric nurses may feel that they don't know enough about to work effectively with.) This is sometimes referred to as the phenomenon of "the unpopular patient."

In theory, such a statement may be true, but the reality is that, except for very rare periods, there's always at least one "problem" or "unpopular" patient on the unit. The idea that everything will be fine once that one particular patient is discharged almost always proves to be an illusion, as another difficult patient soon pops up to take his or her place.

All nurses can do is to provide the best care possible to whoever is on their unit on a given day and try not to get caught up with angry feelings that their colleagues may have about one particular patient being there, as that only makes things worse.

Sketch # 21

Besides The Prof, there were two other psychiatrists on the unit, each having weekly patient rounds. In one of these rounds, I gave a report on a particular patient's status. The patient had been admitted two weeks previously with a diagnosis of manic depression. I stated that he appeared to have slept well, with no evidence of any psychotic thinking, no agitated behavior, no elevated or depressed mood, and so forth. After I had given my nursing report, the patient came into the room, and when asked by the psychiatrist about these issues, he contradicted exactly everything I had said. He complained of not being able to sleep well, of feeling that he was going to "explode" all of the time, and of sometimes hearing voices.

I felt humiliated. It was as if, in front of the whole treatment team with additional medical students, I had just made up an entirely erroneously report and made a fool of myself.

I had interacted with the patient on many occasions over the previous week, I had carefully read the notes written by other staff members in his medical record and was therefore pretty confident that my report was an accurate one. Yet I ended up feeling totally embarrassed.

The psychiatrist may have noted my discomfort, as he then turned to the group of medical students and said to them: "This is a good example of a patient saying quite different things to a doctor than he or she does to other people. It's not uncommon, as patients know that it's the doctor who has the power to discharge them or keep them in hospital, prescribe them medication or not, and that will often affect what they tell us as opposed to what they tell other staff."

Thought: As I was to discover over the rest of my career, the doctor was right. Patients do view the different members of their treatment team differently, not only in terms how much they may individually have learned to trust them, but also in the broader sense of how much power over their lives they see each team member as having.

Nursing staff members are usually seen by patients as being the people who have power over their minute-by-minute everyday lives. Nursing staff get them up in the morning, tell them when to go to groups or other activities, tell them when to eat, when to turn off the TV at night, and when to go to bed. Nursing staff also intervene when any unsafe behaviors break out and make decisions about any conflicts between patients. So, on an ongoing basis, patients view nursing staff members as the people who have power over the quality of their everyday life, even while that view may well be impacted by psychotic thinking.

So, what patients say to nursing staff will at times be colored by that perception of them, and similarly what they say to doctors may be colored by their perception that the doctors have the power to discharge them, prescribe medications, and make recommendations and reports to a judge.

In the case above, the patient had some legal issues stemming from his behaviors when in a manic phase, and it appeared that he was regarding it as being in his best interest to remain in hospital at that time. This consideration affected his self-report to the psychiatrist.

Sketch # 22

While I was at this hospital I wrote some articles that were published in the now-defunct magazine, *Nursing Mirror*, then the competitor of the *Nursing Times*.

Of the two magazines, the *Mirror* had a reputation for being more interested in psychiatric nursing than the *Times*, and it was also more sympathetic to the unionization of nursing staff members with other health staff members, while the *Times* was allied to the Royal College of Nursing.

Over the next six years I had a total of five such articles published, all related to clinical issues that I had observed on units on which I was working as a staff nurse.

I was paid either twenty or forty pounds for each one, depending upon word count; both decent sums of money to me at that time.

Thought: A teaching hospital where a clinical and academic culture of clinical observation and exploration exists and is actively encouraged is an ideal environment for a nurse to come up with topics to write an article about, no matter how modest they may be (as mine were.)

Nurses should look out for anything in their clinical work that catches their eye as being particularly interesting or something that they hadn't thought about before, because if it's attracted their interest, it may well be of interest to other nurses as well.

And nurses who find something they think might make a publishable article should not keep putting off writing, although they might find it very easy to come up with multiple reasons not to start working, as it takes time and effort to write one.

For my experience was that my enthusiasm for writing articles, and quite probably my creative abilities, lasted for only a relatively short period.

Later in my career, I would write small articles for hospital newsletters, and would periodically write letters to various psychiatric publications, but my urge and ability to write articles for national professional magazines did dwindle away, so I would encourage any nurse to get writing while his or her enthusiasm and creativity to do so exist.

Sketch # 23

Some years later, I learned that the unit had closed following a series of patient suicides by defenestration, meaning jumping out of a high window.

General hospital staff members usually tend not to look upon psychiatric units in their midst particularly favorably, so when this unit opened it was placed on the top fifth floor, as far away from the rest of the hospital units as possible. But as it turned out, the physical features of the unit were not completely modified to accommodate a psychiatric population in total safety.

The end result was that some small windows in the patients' rooms could still be opened. They were small enough that no one believed that it would be possible for anyone to squeeze through them, yet after a few years, one determined suicidal patient eventually saw the possibility there, somehow got through, and fell to his death. Another two later followed before the problem could be fixed.

Thought: Psychiatric nurses always emphasize to their patients that they are safe when they are in an inpatient unit, but everyone knows that there is an element of myth in this—and no one talks about that. Nurses must find the unsafe features of their areas—and they will always be there—before a patient finds them.

Suicide attempts, like escape attempts, often occur in copycat fashion on psychiatric units, as other patients see that what they had previously regarded as being impossible to do are actually possible. So all workers must practice vigilance at the highest level, especially immediately after a suicide or escape attempt.

CHAPTER 3

A Caribbean Hospital

After a year at the midlands hospital, I again got the itch to travel, and in the old *Nursing Mirror* journal, I saw an advert for nurses to work at a hospital in Bermuda. That fitted my bill exactly, so off I went.

I lived in a nurse's home shared by the hospital and the island's general hospital, next to the botanical gardens, just as beautiful a place as anyone could have wished for.

The units at the hospital were arranged as quadrangles, with single-patient rooms on each corridor and an open grassy area in the middle.

On the evening shift, most patients usually drifted back to their rooms after the eight o'clock medication pass and stayed there until breakfast the next morning. It's a routine familiar to psychiatric nurses the whole world over. It became my habit to go round to each patient room at that time, asking patients how they were doing, trying to engage them in some conversation. Usually most patients didn't want to talk, but on any given evening one or two did.

In 1975, it was considered to be safe for a psychiatric nurse to talk with patients in their rooms as long as the door was open, so this is what I would do. In fact, we were taught that the best seating arrangement in the patient's room was to have the patient sitting next to the door so that he or she could get out quickly should they start to become anxious. The staff member would be the person sitting further into the room.

Over the years, this protocol has changed significantly, as staff member safety became recognized as an important issue, with advice regarding the safest seating arrangement for a staff member talking to a patient in his or her room then being changed so that the staff member sits in the seat closest to the door so that he or she can escape quickly if feeling in danger.

In our current era, staff members are advised never to talk with patients in their rooms, even with the door open. Rather, staff members should talk with patients in a quiet area on the unit, usually where they can be seen from the nursing station.

Sketch # 24

Mr. G. had been admitted to the hospital after his parents had expressed concern that he was steadily becoming "different" from the son they had previously known. He was twenty-three years old and had become more and more isolative, secretive, and anxious. But there were no obvious psychotic symptoms, so no one really knew what was going on with him.

And after three weeks on the unit, we knew nothing more about him. Other than coming out for meals, he stayed in his room and was rather furtive and anxious when staff members tried to talk to him. On my evening rounds of the unit, he always avoided talking to me.

So it was therefore somewhat of a surprise to me when, one evening, he asked me to sit down and talk to him. He started by saying that, before he said anything, he needed me to promise that I wouldn't repeat what he was going to say to anyone else.

My reply was the reply that every psychiatric nurse must give when a patient makes that condition: "I'm very interested in what you have to say, but I'm sorry—if what you say may affect your treatment, then I will have to let the other treatment team members know about it." (See Sketch # 42.) He paused for a few seconds, considering what to do, but in the end the possibility of relieving the burden of his thoughts won out over his paranoia, and he started to talk.

Wonderful and Weird

Hesitatingly, he talked about his increasing anxiety that somehow a chip had been inserted into his brain, and that messages and instructions were being transmitted to him through this chip. He believed that these messages were most likely coming from a satellite in outer space. He didn't know who had inserted the chip, but he believed that the person or organization was now in control of his life. He asked if the chip could be removed so that he could regain control of his life.

As he talked, I almost had to catch myself from crying. For, in the absence of any other signs or symptoms, we had been coming to the conclusion that he must be in some sort of youthful life crisis rather than an actual illness. But now it was clear that he had a serious psychotic illness, most likely paranoid schizophrenia. And having schizophrenia meant that he probably would never fall in love or have any other rich emotional relationships or friendships. He would most likely not have a meaningful job that would last longer than a very brief period. In other words, he was a young man who would most likely have none of the wonderful experiences that the rest of us take for granted. Instead, he would have a life of constant anxiety and fear, tormented by thoughts and hallucinations that he would be unable to control. His parents would take him home and encourage him to take his medications, but after a while he would refuse and maybe start to threaten them, and then be readmitted to the hospital. And that would be the pattern of his life.

In psychiatry, we try to be very optimistic about serious mental illnesses such as schizophrenia. That helps to give hope to our patients as well as hope to ourselves. And it also gives hope to politicians who might otherwise view psychiatric patients as being only a life-long drain on the public treasury. But even after several generations of increasingly sophisticated medications, schizophrenia remains an illness that confounds any attempt at curing it.

Other than my last talk with my father, I think that the conversation with Mr. G. was the saddest one I ever had.

Thought: Psychiatric nurses must carefully persist with their patients, even when there is little hope that their interest in them will lead anywhere positive. This patient was developing schizophrenia whether we discovered it during this admission, or it became obvious later on. But it is now well proven that, if we can start treating patients during their first psychotic episode, we have a good chance of at least softening the impact of their illness over the course of their lives, and hopefully that was the case here.

Sketch # 25

No matter how beautiful it is, Bermuda is still a small island, and Bermudians will tell newcomers that they will become stir-crazy unless they get off it every now and then.

So, I took a vacation to Jamaica, figuring that I might never have another chance in my life to do so. My imagination had often taken me to Jamaica, going back to my boyhood obsession with collecting stamps and fantasizing about the countries that the stamps came from.

While I was in Kingston, the capital of Jamaica, I was interested to see what their psychiatric hospital was like, so I planned a visit. The administration kindly allowed me to go onto one of the wards there and talk to the nurse in charge. She was cheerful yet stoic, spending most of her shift giving out medications to the seventy patients in her care, with only two nursing assistants to help her with everything.

Patients had rooms on three sides of the ward, but the fourth side led directly to the Caribbean Sea. She said that it was originally built that way as many Jamaicans didn't swim well, so the sea was considered an effective barrier. I asked if patients, nevertheless, ever tried to escape by swimming away. She said that sometimes they did, and also said that they occasionally had a suicide by drowning.

I asked her what the main illnesses were that they were treating on her ward, expecting her to list schizophrenia and manic depression. I was therefore greatly surprised when she said that the most prevalent diagnosis on her unit was marijuana-induced psychosis.

I knew that marijuana certainly resulted in problematic distortions of perception and judgement, but I had never heard of it resulting in a psychosis before. When I asked her to talk more about it, she explained it in this way: "In other countries people take marijuana in order to relax, feel sexy, that sort of thing. But here in Jamaica young men who are Rastafarians take ganja in order to be able to speak directly with their God, Jah. And once they start speaking to God, that takes things to a quite different level. They then sometimes lose control of their thinking and become psychotic."

She said that usually they recovered and were able to be discharged after a few weeks, but that some remained psychotic permanently.

Thought: In a substance-abuse course that I later took at a Boston university, the teacher emphasized that "set and setting" (i.e., who you're with and why you're doing what you're doing) were the most important factors in determining someone's individual response to taking drugs, and this culturally different effect of taking marijuana seems to support that idea.

Sketch # 26

Paradise or not, there were some social and political tensions in Bermuda as a whole at this time, and these tensions inevitably were reflected in the nursing group working at the hospital. Racial tensions were one of the issues, but the main tension was between native Bermudians and nonnative people there on work permits. This revolved around the fear of native Bermudians that nonnatives might end up buying much of the limited real estate on the island, so a variety of measures had been put in place to help prevent this. One of these was that nonnatives had to be resident on the island at least for one year before they could buy property, so nurses coming from Britain or the Caribbean to work at the hospital were routinely only given a one-year contract, after which they had to leave the island.

Whenever serious tensions occur in a nursing staff, then cliques inevitably develop, and patient care equally starts to deteriorate as patient cliques paralleling those of the staff also then start to develop.

Aware of this, nursing management looked for ways to proactively resolve any divisions in the nursing staff before the situation started to impact patient care. To do this they established a psycho-dynamically oriented weekly group led by a psychologist, with nurses being strongly encouraged to attend without attendance actually being mandatory. The idea was that, as staff members got to know and understand each other on a personal basis—rather than each member representing a rival social and political viewpoints—then they would become a cohesive work group rather than a divided one.

It was a well-intentioned effort, but a failed one. A number of supervisors and staff nurses attended the group, but even though they were strongly encouraged to do so by the group leader, the supervisors were understandably reluctant to divulge personal data that might become the subject of gossip or be otherwise used against them by line staff members. Some nurses eventually started to talk about personal issues, and these were at times deeply personal ones.

But far from making the group more cohesive, the more personal information that group members disclosed, the more it tended to produce alarm rather than trust in the other members. People started to leave the group, and it eventually was abandoned.

Thought: Getting staff together to openly discuss problems within the group that might be impacting patient care is essential, but doing this in the format of a regular staff meeting is far more likely to be successful than as a psycho-dynamically oriented group such as this one.

Such groups were the fashion of that era, but revealing personal issues, particularly when staff members from different administrative levels were present, did not engender any real trust amongst group members, and whatever divisions there were among staff members pretty much remained as they had been before.

CHAPTER 4

A Boston University

Sketch # 27

At Christmastime, a nurse came to work at the Bermuda hospital during the holiday period. She said that she was a student at the school of nursing at an American university and had come home during the academic breaks to earn money. She told me that, even though I didn't have a bachelor's degree in nursing, since I had a degree in something and was a registered nurse in the UK, I would be able to get into graduate school in the United States. That sounded like an interesting idea, so I applied to several universities and ended up being accepted at a Boston university in their master of psychiatric–adult mental health nursing program, starting in 1977.

As my money was limited, I was very anxious to complete the course on time, so after the daytime lectures were over, I diligently went to the library every evening to read the assigned text books until it closed at ten o'clock. After a few weeks, some concerned classmates convinced me that this level of intensity was not necessary in graduate work, so I started to relax my schedule and hence enjoy the work more.

One of the mandatory courses was "Nursing Theorists," as nursing theory was the hot topic in academic nursing at that time. It was part of the general feminist movement in the predominantly female nursing field, aimed toward gaining professional equality with predominantly male medicine. As part of that general movement, nursing was trying to prove that their training, like that of physicians, properly belonged in universities rather than in hospitals.

And the way that one proved that one belonged in an academic setting was to have a language and a body of knowledge that belonged uniquely to the profession.

Hence, in the 1960s and '70s, there was an explosion of different nursing theories, all designed to establish nursing's academic credentials.

We had a mandatory nursing theory course in which we studied a number of these competing theories. The professor told us that we should "adopt" the one that we liked best, and then use it in our subsequent practices.

Most of the theories appeared to many of my colleagues and to me as just plain silly, no matter how earnestly the professors presented them as legitimate science. Though, oddly enough, the more bizarre the theory, the more adherents it attracted, and adherents quickly became competitively zealous and vocal in defending their chosen theory.

In the big scheme, the era of nursing theories being promulgated as being scientifically valid and valuable to real-life nursing practice was probably a necessary step in the professional growth of nursing. Yet it did alarm me that academic nursing could take them all so seriously when they were clearly pseudoscience at best.

But, at the local level, the university itself couldn't have been too impressed by the academic credentials as presented by these nursing theories, as they closed the school of nursing a few years later.

Thoughts: When I had occasionally wondered where my future career might take me, I had figured that I would probably end up in nursing education. But listening to well-established nursing professors extoling the quality of the emperor's new clothes (the new nursing theories) when we students could see very well for ourselves that the emperor was actually naked, gave me second thoughts about my future lying there.

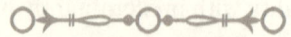

This time period saw the height of psychodynamic psychiatry, and the clinical teaching at the university reflected that. When writing a paper on patients we were working with, we had to emphasize what defense mechanisms they were using, and the status of their object relations, with the clues that these offered the nurse regarding identifying the patients' diagnoses.

I did find this interesting and useful in thinking about a patient's illness. Even though the later era of biological psychiatry basically swept all of this away, and many psychiatric nurses now have little idea what defense mechanisms or object relations are, there may well come a time when they will be worth revisiting.

For whenever I still hear a patient attribute behavior and faults to someone else when they clearly belong to themselves, I still think to myself something like: *That's projection, and that probably means the patient is paranoid.*

Sketch # 28

The clinical rotation that I was assigned to there was the partial hospitalization program at a Boston, Massachusetts, hospital. This was a prestigious, expensive, private teaching hospital, with wonderful old buildings and beautiful landscaping by Frederick Law Olmstead.

During our orientation, it turned out that, a few years before this time, the nursing department at the hospital had officially adopted Ida Orlando's nursing theory model from her book, *The Dynamic Nurse-Patient Relationship* (7), in line with what was expected of nursing departments in academic settings in that period. But I was interested to note that, by the time I went there, nobody was actually practicing it at all anywhere in the hospital inpatient units or clinics. One person in nursing education offered to teach it to someone if he or she showed any interest, but she was basically all that remained of the project after just a short time. This reinforced the opinion that I had already formed at the Boston university regarding the relevance of nursing theory models: they may have some positive role to play in establishing nursing as a legitimate subject for study in universities, but their practical significance for working nurses was very limited at best.

This partial hospital was an outpatient clinic where patients gathered for groups and other programming, and sometimes medications. Patients attended for five days (Monday through Friday) or less, as determined by the acuity of their illness.

I found myself quite unnerved at times by working in an outpatient clinic, as some patients would come in saying they felt that they might kill themselves when they got home. My instinct was to want to immediately hospitalize them, but instead staff members would carry out some intensive assessments, huddle over the results, and then usually the patient would be allowed to go home if he or she gave assurances about personal safety.

Working in an outpatient clinic caused me much more anxiety than working a locked inpatient unit. Not being absolutely sure that patients weren't going to kill themselves when they left the clinic was very uncomfortable to me and caused me some sleepless nights. On inpatient units, there are certainly anxiety-producing events involving patient violence against themselves and others. But staff members nevertheless have a large degree of control over what happens in a locked unit, and they know how to respond to unsafe incidents.

But watching patients leave the clinic without being certain that they would come back the next day was so uncomfortable for me that I knew that my nursing career would be spent on inpatient units from then on. Psychiatric nurses tend to separate themselves this way: some are okay with the uncertainty of not absolutely knowing if their patients are safe or not, and they work in outpatient clinics. Others need to have more certainty, need to feel more in control of situations, and they work at inpatient units, usually locked.

This anxiety on my part turned out to be well worthwhile, though, as I also met my future wife, Karen, there. She was my clinical supervisor.

Thought: Psychiatric nursing isn't just one specialty; it consists of several subspecialties. Nurses must know what they are comfortable in within the field and avoid areas that they are not comfortable with, as otherwise they may not enjoy their work and may not do it well.

CHAPTER 5

A South London Hospital

After graduating from the Boston university, I returned to England and began work in 1978 as a charge nurse (the male equivalent of a sister) at a hospital in south London. It was a small hospital that treated predominantly medical-surgical geriatric patients, but it also supported two psychiatric units.

Sketch # 29

On one of these units a patient was admitted with a diagnosis of paranoid schizophrenia. He was in his mid-fifties and had worked as a sailor on an Australian ship. During a recent voyage to London, he had become psychotic and violent, and had been admitted directly from the ship once it had docked.

He continued to be very paranoid of staff members and patients alike, convinced that someone was going to try to kill him, and periodically he would then attack whoever he thought was the danger to him. In England at that time, the use of mechanical restraints to safely contain violent patient behavior was not generally allowed. So what happened in such cases was that the patient would be wrestled to the ground by staff members and given intramuscular injections of sedative and antipsychotic medications. The patient usually continued to struggle, so staff members would then keep him or her pinned to the ground until the mediation took effect. This would often be twenty to thirty minutes.

One day this patient assaulted another patient as a result of his paranoid delusions, and an emergency injection was ordered for him. I was the nurse who gave him that injection. As we held him on the floor waiting for the medication to take effect, he started to focus on me, threatening to assault me as soon as the opportunity presented itself. And for several days afterward, he would hand me little pieces of paper on which he'd written messages: "I know where you live." "One day I'll be waiting in a dark alley to kill you."

I always made sure that the treatment team members were aware of these threats, and I put the notes in the patient's chart. But I couldn't stop from being quite scared of being focused upon in this way, and of what might happen to me in the future. And even when the patient was discharged, apparently stabilized, and saying that he meant no harm to anyone, I remained very aware of his earlier threats when I was walking about town.

As time went by and nothing happened, I gradually stopped thinking about his threats, but for probably a year after he was discharged, I lived with a certain degree of fear.

Thoughts: Nurses must always take patient threats seriously—always. They're part of the job for psychiatric nurses, and while they fairly soon learn to live their lives without excessive fear of these threats, they must never just tell themselves that they're nothing to worry about, because sometimes they are. Nurses must make sure that their supervisors and the treatment team members know that they have been threatened, and make sure that the threat has been documented. Talking with other staff members who have themselves been the subject of threats also helps to make the experience more manageable. In many US states these days there are also often "duty to protect" forms that staff members should fill out when they are directly threatened by a patient.

Sketch # 30

The hospital's medical specialty was chronic respiratory illnesses, and one of the few remaining units of "iron lung" patients was located there, catering mainly to patients whose breathing had been impaired by polio. Every summer a party was held on the small hospital lawn for these patients and also those who were using cuirass shells to breathe. (This shell is attached to a power unit and worn around the patient's body. By manipulating the diaphragm, the shell actively controls both phases of the respiratory cycle.)

The iron lungs, each with a patient inside, were carefully wheeled out onto the hospital lawn, there to feel the sun on their faces for the first time in a year. Tea and cake were served.

It was a surreal sight, those couple of hours—those weird contraptions, looking more like coffins than life-maintaining medical equipment, with their hundreds of yards of electric wires strung around the lawn, and the cheerful nurses bustling about, sometimes tripping over them.

Patients in their iron lungs appeared to enjoy it all, though there was also some element of relief when they returned to the unit, as they were always acutely vigilant in making sure that their machines were plugged in properly, for electrical current was a matter of life or death to them.

Thought: Patients with serious chronic illnesses, medical or psychiatric, and the nurses who care for them, need things to look forward to and get excited about. Even just planning and making happen a yearly two-hour break in the battle went a long way for both the patients and nurses.

Sketch # 31

By 1979, the political pendulum was beginning to swing away from the militant left-wing focus of the previous decade, but there was still life left in it. There was a union call for one-day industrial action nationally in the National Health Service, focusing largely on low wages, and the union branch at my hospital decided to participate in this.

We carefully made sure that all of the units had their regular staffing, and we got approval from the police for a march. We drew the hospital's and union's names on a bed sheet, and with that as our banner, marched up and down the high street for about an hour chanting slogans. At the end, some of us went to the pub to celebrate while others prepared to go to work for the next shift. We were exhilarated because we had "done something," though we also knew that what we had actually achieved was probably quite minimal.

Thoughts: My overall experience has been that the very best working environment for nurses is to be found in nonunionized, not-for-profit, academically affiliated private hospitals. In those, a wise management has the resources to usually avoid seriously antagonizing its nurses while providing many professional and academic opportunities valuable to them. In that scenario, having a nurse's union serves only to inevitably introduce a political agenda, which eventually erodes the professional potential of their work.

On the other hand, where public hospitals (the National Health Service in the UK, and federal, state, and county hospitals in the United States) are concerned, however, my experience has been that unions representing nurses are necessary because those organizations are run by regularly changing political appointees who, in turn, have political agendas, and who rarely hesitate to place their political goals above the best interests of the health systems that they run. In that scenario, nurses need to have some protection from the inevitable vagaries of these political appointees. And unions can do this—sometimes well, sometimes badly.

Nurses who work in psychiatric public hospitals with virtually no academic affiliations have my deepest admiration. They know that they are working in systems where money and marginal staffing will be never-ending issues. They know that they will be caring for the acute, often violent, long-term patients whom private hospitals have the luxury of refusing to admit. They know that they will get little training other than the excruciating annual mandatory classes. And they can pretty much forget about any professional conferences. Yet knowing all of this, day after day, year after year, these nurses turn up at the start of their shifts, and for the next eight hours, care for their patients in the most professional manner that they can. In such settings, some nurses do allow their professionalism to deteriorate, but every state hospital in the United States has its cadre of true salt-of-the-earth nurses without whom the hospital simply could not operate.

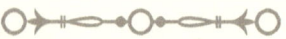

This hospital closed in 1997.

CHAPTER 6

A Central London Hospital

Sketch # 32

In 1980 my heart was telling me that I needed to go back to the United States. Karen and I had been in communication since I had left Boston, but it was clear to me that I needed to go back permanently if our relationship was going to go the way I dearly wanted it to go. But in order to do that, I had to first become registered in general as well as psychiatric nursing, so I entered the Nightingale Training School for Nurses in London. I was always interested in history, and I loved being able to train in the first school of nursing in the world founded by Florence in 1860.

I also loved being able to live in the nurses' home, with its direct view over Westminster Bridge to Big Ben and Parliament. I said to myself that, no matter where I might live for the rest of my life, I would never have a more glamorous view to wake up to each morning.

Yet, after six months of being awakened in the middle of the night by Big Ben striking every quarter of an hour, I was content to move to another nurses' home in Westminster. From there I walked by Scotland Yard, Westminster Abbey, Parliament and Big Ben, and over Westminster or Lambeth Bridge on my way to work every day. Twice while I was walking to work, the queen drove past me on Victoria Street in her ceremonial horses and carriage on her way back to Buckingham Palace having met a foreign head of state at Victoria Station.

General nursing wasn't the nursing that I wanted to be doing long term, but everything at the hospital was of a high quality, and all of my colleagues were smart and warm hearted, so it was very easy and enjoyable working here.

Some of the hospital wards were still based in old Victorian buildings designed by Florence Nightingale herself. One such was the male urology ward, dubbed "The Rubber Jungle" by nurses throughout the hospital. The ward sister was an old German nurse who proudly stuck to the Nightingale traditions of the hospital. Thus, she started the day by gathering all of the staff members at one end of the ward to say prayers, in which many patients also joined. After that, nurses were ordered to open the small top windows to ventilate the ward with fresh river air. We could just see Florence smiling in approval, as she was a real stickler for ventilation.

Sir A. F., a celebrated ballet choreographer, was a patient on this ward while I was working there. A steady succession of senior hospital administrators came onto the ward to welcome him, enquire solicitously about his health and whether he was satisfied with the care being provided. He greeted them all very graciously, but in a quiet moment slyly asked me the rhetorical question: "How often do you see them up here when there's not a well-known person lying in one of your beds?"

On New Year's Eve night, the emergency room and many of the hospital's corridors were lined solidly with gurneys, each with someone sleeping off his or her earlier revelries in Trafalgar Square. By daybreak most had awoken and sheepishly gone on their way.

In obstetrics, I saw my first birth, and like many before me shed a tear or two. Elizabeth was her name. Not quite as beautiful as my own daughter, Hilary, was when she was born, but close! The obstetrics sister was determined to prove that her department was not laggardly on the hot topic issue of gender equality, and proudly told me that, in Elizabeth's case, I had become the first male nurse at the hospital to perform a pre-delivery pubic shave!

In pediatrics, I worked with a delightful three-year-old girl diagnosed with tuberous sclerosis, who had a few weeks to live. I'm okay with violent, suicidal, or regressed psychiatric patients, but as most psychiatric nurses will say, don't ask me to work with dying children again.

At that time, student nurses in their last year of training acted in the charge nurse role on the night shift, and I had that rotation on a medical-surgical ward. I remember constantly and earnestly hoping that no medical emergency would break out on my shift, as I was far from certain that I knew enough to handle one appropriately. Fortunately for me, my hopes were realized.

We finished the training with our national exams, consisting of morning and afternoon sessions over two days. After the morning sessions, we walked down to The Pineapple pub and had a couple of pints while playing "Pressure" by David Bowie and Queen over and over again on the jukebox. We then trooped back to the hospital just in time for the afternoon exam. That was 1982, but I probably wouldn't be advising anyone now to be drinking alcohol between exams!

I had a rotation on the night shift in the emergency room (ER), and there I did my first real CPR—on a fifty-year-old man who had a cardiac arrest. I completely forgot the formal CPR protocol in my haste, and in my anxiety succeeded in breaking two of his ribs. But he did live!

I also stitched up a long scalp wound sustained by a character well known to the regular emergency room staff, who had fallen down in the street when drunk. Technically I shouldn't have done the stitching, but the resident doctor on duty was tired and asked me if I wanted to try my hand at it, which I did!

During this rotation, I couldn't help but notice that the regular ER nursing and medical staff didn't really like having psychiatric patients in the ER very much. And that also went for the ERs in the other general hospitals that I was familiar with.

The reasons for this were varied and often had a legitimate basis. Psychiatric patients that were loud, exhibited bizarre behaviors, or were unable to follow directions to sit quietly until they could be attended to really could disrupt the whole ER and make a lot more work for the staff. In the case of potentially violent patients, staff members simply feared for their own safety. Trying to effectively treat acutely ill psychiatric patients who deny being ill or needing treatment is also very frustrating to those not used to it.

But even if the ER was relatively quiet and the staffing level wasn't an issue, the nurses and doctors on duty would sometimes groan a little when a patient who had made a suicide attempt came in, and particularly so with self-injurious behaviors that had no actual suicidal intent. At first, I couldn't understand this, as many people have had suicidal thoughts at some point in their lives, or have family members, friends, or neighbors who have made suicidal attempts, so I assumed that there would always be some empathy for suicidal patients.

But sometimes there would not only not be empathy, there would be actual anger toward these patients, sometimes thinly disguised anger, particularly if this was not the first time that a patient had come to the ER following a suicide or self-injurious attempt. I knew of a case at another hospital where the ER doctor treating a sixteen-year-old girl who had overdosed following a fight with her boyfriend was clearly angered by the situation and told the nurse to get the largest gastric tube she could find for the stomach pumping procedure. When she asked why, the doctor replied that, if the treatment was unpleasant for the patient, she might think twice before taking another overdose after the next fight.

ER nurses often make no secret of this this dislike, giving as their chief reason for it that the ER should be primarily for patients who have become desperately ill for reasons beyond their control, and that patients who have deliberately inflicted injuries upon themselves simply take valuable time away from this primary mission (8).

Thoughts: The feelings that psychiatric patients bring up in ER staff members are essentially the same feelings that psychiatric nurses have to resolve in their own work. We all have a frustrating sense of helplessness when, no matter what good nursing care and good medical treatment patients receive, they may be soon repeating the same pathological behaviors. Psychiatric nurses must eventually understand that this is just how many mental illnesses go—including denial of illness and refusal to take medications—but it is easy to see why this patient behavior may sometimes be seen by nurses in other specialties as being willful and infuriating.

Nurses see themselves as in the business of healing people. The unspoken deal here is that they do their best nursing bit and patients, in response, do their bit by being healed and staying healed. But when patients keep coming back with the same signs and symptoms, then the deal is broken and nurses can feel helpless. They are doing their bit, so why don't the patients do theirs? And that helplessness can easily lead to frustration and then anger.

It's that stage of anger that nurses have to avoid reaching, as then they have the potential to start behaving unprofessionally. Nurses avoid that anger by understanding that no one is immune to it and that it's a good idea to talk about it with colleagues when they recognize it in themselves. And, nurses should talk about it with colleagues when they recognize it in them.

Sketch # 33

I went to a lecture by Dr. S. W., presented at the hospital. He had run psychiatry at the hospital from the late 1940s through the early 1970s but had been retired for some years. He had always been a fierce advocate of medical model psychiatry and talked with relish of his heated debates in the 1930s with psychoanalyst Helene Deutsch.

He remained an advocate of treatments such as psychosurgery, insulin shock therapy, and deep sleep therapy, but was particularly passionate in his belief that electroconvulsive therapy (ECT) remained the single most effective treatment for depression and mania. In the manner that made him a controversial figure in his time, he stated that ECT was most effective when given to a patient in deep sleep, and that in the 1950s he had performed this with patients without telling them beforehand what he was going to do. He almost seemed to regret that ethical considerations would now exclude such practices.

Thoughts: I liked and respected Dr. W. In an age when millions of people with psychotic illnesses were languishing basically untreated in gigantic psychiatric hospitals with patient populations the size of small towns (for example, a state hospital in Georgia housed 10,000 patients in the 1940s), he and others like him at least tried to develop concrete methods of helping them, even if his approach was at times reckless.

Psychoanalysis was and remains a culturally celebrated treatment for neurotic patients who can financially afford it, but psychoanalysis never interested itself in those millions of patients in the huge psychiatric hospitals of the world, and never did anything for them.

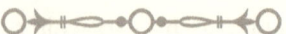

When I started working at my first hospital, there were several older nurses who had been involved in giving patients insulin shock therapy. They all said that, while the treatment was potentially a dangerous one, in their experience it did have positive effects for patients with schizophrenia. A very smart veteran psychiatrist once told me that insulin therapy was one of the old treatments well worth a second look if the political environment ever allowed it.

Sketch # 34

During my post registration period at the hospital, I had a rotation at the south London hospital where I had previously worked in the psychiatric services, only now I was working on the respiratory unit with "iron lung" patients (see Sketch # 29.)

These were patients with virtually no control over their bodies, and therefore were totally dependent upon nurses doing pretty much everything for them. This intense nurse-patient relationship produced some consistent themes of passive aggression, in which the patients struggled to gain control of something in their lives while nurses tried to allow them to do this without feeling manipulated (9).

Ms. J. was the dominant personality on the unit. An intelligent woman, she had contracted polio when she was four years old and subsequently developed scoliosis. Now thirty-three years old, she had been on the unit in an iron lung for five years, with little chance for change in sight. The only control she had over her body was talking and making some minor movements in her arms and hands.

This was a scenario in which anyone would think that all nurses, full of empathy for the unenviable circumstances that the patient found herself in, would be wholeheartedly throwing themselves into Ms. J's care.

And while that was certainly true, it was also true that staff coffee breaks and change-of-shift reports were often filled with complaints about Ms. J. and how difficult it was to look after her. The main complaint was that she was constantly putting them in no-win situations no matter what they did, and that they ended up feeling either frustrated or guilty after caring for her. Neither of these was a desirable option.

For instance, Ms. J. would ring her bell for a nurse with some minor request. When this request was met, her bell would soon ring again with another minor request. And so it would go. Often the requests were phrased in an indirect manner, such as saying to the nurse, "I wonder if there's any bread left in the kitchen." What she was really wanted was for the nurse to make her a sandwich.

To Ms. J., the frequency and nature interactions with the nurses were just about the only things that she could control in her life, but to the nurses, on some days, her behavior was seen as plain passive-aggressive manipulation that left them frustrated and angry.

Sometimes a nurse would say to her, "Why not think up a list of things that you need me to do so you don't need to ring the bell so often?" Or, "Please just tell me what you want instead of making me have to try to guess what it is." Her response to these sorts of comments was consistently a variation of, "You wouldn't say that to me if I wasn't a cripple!" And this would inevitably evoke guilt in the nurse.

Faced with guilt if they didn't do exactly what Ms. J. wanted, how and when she wanted it, the nurses ended up opting to simply follow her instructions while seething about it inside and waiting for the next coffee break to vent about it.

Thoughts: The patients on this unit were certainly a unique group, but passive-aggressive behaviors are common with anyone who feels that he or she has no direct control over a situation and is angry about that. These people therefore seek to assert some indirect control, and in the process often end up reflecting their own anger in someone else.

Thus, passive-aggressive behaviors are not uncommon with involuntary patients on a psychiatric unit who are angry about being there, and they may sometimes use these techniques with psychiatric staff. For instance, if a staff member is annoyed with a particular patient for any reason and that patient then asks to be legitimately let off the unit, the staff member may make him or her wait a minute or two longer than necessary before opening the door, probably causing the patient to become angry.

The ability to withhold something is a characteristic of many passive-aggressive behaviors, such as withholding the quick opening of the unit door in the previous example. Withholding information from a colleague may be another form of passive-aggression on a unit.

Being polite and speaking directly to people is the simple way to avoid getting in passive-aggressive games on your unit.

CHAPTER 7

A Boston, Massachusetts, State Hospital

Sketch # 35

I returned to Boston, Massachusetts, and did the state nursing exams there in 1983.

Having worked in the National Health Service in England, I was familiar with public health systems, and that led me to apply for a job as a staff nurse at a state hospital in Boston. The nursing administrators there said that they would apply for a two-year work visa for me, an application that would certainly succeed, they assured me.

But rather than wait until the visa was actually approved, they asked if I would work as a nurse at the hospital pending that approval, as they were critically short of nurses. The idea was that I would not be paid until the visa was formally approved, at which point I would be formally put on the payroll and then get the back pay I was due.

I wasn't sure of the legality of working with patients as a registered nurse without actually having a contract, but I was assured that it wasn't a problem, and I was just excited to be working in the United States, so I agreed.

This hospital had a long and excellent reputation as a treatment and teaching hospital, but at the time that I joined them, the glory days were long gone. A general air of chaos now pervaded. There were few professional permanent staff there, while patients were automatically admitted "off the street" upon request of the police or emergency room physicians. When I came onto my unit at the start of the first shift, it was routine the find patients who had been admitted during the previous night sleeping on couches and chairs in the day room, as there simply weren't enough beds for everyone.

The main door to the unit was not locked, as the official Department of Mental Health protocol of the time was that, since psychiatric treatments were effective, and patients were therefore eagerly seeking to take advantage of these treatments, locked doors were no longer necessary. Having locked doors was also believed to further serve to perpetuate the idea that all psychiatric patients were dangerous and needed to be locked up.

Reality did not match this optimistic policy, however. So, in order to avoid a mass exodus of patients from the unit, the physically strongest male staff members were assigned by the hour to stand by the door in order to prevent any patient who wanted to leave from actually doing so. I couldn't help but think of Cerberus in Dante's *Inferno*.

The day room was usually filled with patients intently staring at the door, knowing that it was open, and simply waiting for an opportunity to run through it. Every now and then, a single patient would charge the door in an escape attempt, and a physical struggle would then ensue with the staff member guarding the door, with other staff members becoming involved as necessary.

Thoughts: Involuntary psychiatric patients almost never want to be in the hospital, and repeatedly ask to be discharged. And every psychiatric nurse has wondered at some point why these patients don't just band together, overpower the staff, take their keys, and escape. The night shift, often minimally staffed with older women, would appear particularly vulnerable to such an event.

Yet it never happens. Why? Psycho-dynamic theorists might speculate that, unconsciously, patients know that they need treatment and should stay in hospital to receive it, no matter how vigorously they may verbally proclaim the opposite. But the most likely explanations to me are: One, acutely psychotic patients are simply too disorganized in their thinking to be able to work cooperatively with one another in any effective manner. And two, paranoid people simply cannot trust anyone else enough to formulate and follow through in any plans with them.

I should add that, while this may be true of a regular psychiatric patient population, it would not necessarily be true of a patient population that includes people with strong anti-social personality disorder (psychopathic) traits, such as forensic psychiatric populations. For these are people who can work effectively together and can even involve psychotic patients in their plans. Nurses working with these populations will find reading *Games Criminals Play* by Bud Allen (10) very helpful in terms of maintaining effective professional boundaries and recognizing dangerous patient strategies.

And as a note to political policy makers: please check out how your policies are working out in practice before you declare great advances in the care of patients in your hospitals.

Sketch # 36

A young woman was admitted one day after getting into a fight with Boston police personnel. She was manic, hadn't slept for days, had thoughts just flying around inside her head, and was in a dysphoric, angry mood.

As an emergency measure, she was ordered to have electroconvulsive therapy (ECT), an excellent treatment for quickly bringing down the agitation level of very manic patients.

But ECT wasn't done at the hospital itself; it was done at a private general hospital perhaps a quarter of a mile away. Since money was always an issue, and the other facility was fairly close, it was decided not to take her there by ambulance, which would be the normal way of taking a patient to another hospital.

Instead, she was mechanically restrained onto a gurney. Escorted by a state policeman with a gun at his side, a mental health worker and I pushed her down the sidewalk of Brookline Avenue with a view of Fenway Park in the distance. Manic to start with and now also quite over stimulated, she thrashed wildly about on the gurney, several times nearly turning it over, while screaming, spitting, swearing, and threatening anyone who came in her line of vision. Pedestrians on the street stopped and stared at us as we went by, and astonished drivers slowed down to see what the commotion was all about.

Privacy issues aside, I couldn't help thinking that, if anything was going to reinforce any public stereotype of psychiatric patients as being dangerous, frothing-at-the-mouth lunatics, that ten-minute walk was it.

The return journey was uneventful, as the general hospital sent her back in an ambulance.

After seven weeks of working at this hospital I was told that my work visa application had been rejected on the grounds that a two-year contract was too long to offer an alien. I asked if I was going to get paid for the time I had worked there as a staff nurse but was told that I wouldn't as I was never legally an employee and therefore not in the payroll system.

Thoughts: ECT really is an effective treatment for some mood disorders, despite the bad reputation that even now continues to surround it. That reputation came about when it was unsuccessfully used to treat psychotic thought disorders such as schizophrenia in the 1940s and '50 s, and was then portrayed in the politically radical 1960s as an example of medical and social oppression of the mentally ill. But for the right patients it remains one of psychiatry's few "wonder" treatments.

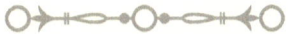

And I learned I should never work without a signed contract in hand!

Malcolm King, RN; MS; CS

The fact that the hospital's nursing administrators had misled me about the legality of my working without a work visa and of being paid retrospectively for my working as a staff nurse there gave me a good idea of the potential problems of running a public health psychiatric hospital in the United States.

This hospital was closed as an inpatient facility in 2003.

CHAPTER 8

A Private Boston Hospital

Sketch # 37

I was told in the decision letter from Immigration that I now had three weeks to leave the country. So Karen and I got married at Boston City Hall, and in 1983 I went to work as a staff nurse at another Boston hospital, the one where I had done my graduate clinical rotation.

This was a grand old private teaching hospital dating back to 1811, full of smart, dedicated people. It had opened the first training school for specifically psychiatric nurses in 1882, and although that had long since closed, the hospital remained a great place to learn the fundamentals of psychiatric nursing.

At this time, the hospital was still predominantly psychodynamic in its treatment philosophy, but biological psychiatry had a solid toehold and was expanding quickly. Unlike many psychiatric units in that era, the doors of this hospital's units were locked, probably due to it being, as a private hospital, very sensitive to the legal and financial risk-management issues related to patient safety.

The beds were always pretty much full with either private-pay patients or folks with good insurance, but as the decade went on and insurance companies started to refuse to pay for many non-biological treatments, the hospital entered a protracted existential crisis, which was experienced by many psychiatric hospitals at that time.

The nursing and other clinical staff members were generally as good as they come, attracted by the reputation of the hospital. As a staff nurse, I found myself particularly interested in the direct-care staff, the mental health workers, as they can play a large part in making a unit a great one or a poor one.

The mental health workers at the hospital were a diverse group. There was a sizeable number of young would-be professionals, earning money and gaining clinical experience as they worked on getting their nursing, social work, or psychology degrees and licenses. But the most interesting group to me consisted of a sizable group of smart, underachieving men in their thirties and forties who had been doing the job for years and, though they complained a lot about it, rarely had concrete plans to do anything different. They knew their job by heart and were very good at it when they wanted to be, but also could be lackadaisical when they didn't want to be good. They liked being part of an intellectually stimulating environment, but for whatever reason, seemed to be unable to take advantage of it in terms of making progress in their own work lives and careers. Their preferred shift note in the patient's medical record was "Quo," it being deemed not cool to write even the modest entry, "Status quo." There were many fascinating, though often infuriating, characters in that group, and I remember them well.

The hospital's campus had been designed after the invention of the telephone, and broke new ground at the time by locating patients in many different "houses" scattered over the campus, which could communicate with each other by using the new invention, rather than having the traditional single huge building where communication was done by walking and talking.

At this time, there was a central dining room, so patients from the various houses were taken through a series of underground tunnels to the dining room for their meals. The tunnels were large enough and reasonably well lit, but they were definitely a little creepy to walk through. One staff member would lead the patient group through the tunnels, and another would bring up the rear to make sure that no one tried to break away.

There were certainly opportunities to escape in the tunnels, but everyone believed that it was impossible to do so, so there were surprisingly few attempts—another of those cases in which most patients buy into a staff-reinforced myth, and everything then goes well.

Years later, a new central dining area was built, the difference this time being that staff and patients ate there at the same time. This was the cause of considerable debate at the time, with staff members of many disciplines preferring not to eat with patients at a nearby table. Being overheard during a clinical discussion was the main objection voiced, but this reasonable objection may well have disguised a simple desire not to be with patients when not actively at work. Medical director Dr. F. S. recognized that the hospital needed to grow beyond its image of class privilege if it was going to financially survive, and that staff and patients eating together was an important metaphor for the changes that would be necessary. So everyone ate at the new dining building, and everything went just fine.

Thought: Nurses who have an opportunity to work at a great teaching hospital should take advantage, even if it's not forever. They'll learn processes from the institution and wisdom from remarkable people, knowledge that will last a lifetime. And they'll learn how to do things well. They'll see what is possible, which will help them to not automatically accept lowering the bar too far when they work at another hospital that may not have the resources of a big teaching hospital.

One of the many remarkable characters here was psychiatrist P. S., who was notorious amongst the nursing staff for conducting at least two, and possibly three, phone calls simultaneously once he had sat down at a table on the unit. This was long before cell phones appeared on the scene, so he would just grab as many phones as he could in that area and start making his calls. This could sometimes be annoying to the nurses who needed those same phones for their own work, but on the whole, it was accepted simply as the price we paid for working with a talented, eccentric colleague. One day on the unit the conversation got around to why Americans tended to be boisterous and outgoing compared to the English, who seem more reserved and quiet. He put down his phones for a few seconds to comment: "Most of the manics left England long ago to emigrate to America, leaving only the schizoid personalities in England." This was one of those things that the smart people in academic settings can come up with, and which give one pause for thought, even if it's theoretically easy enough to poke holes in.

Sketch # 38

I started working on a locked male-female unit. The average length of stay was measured in months, but in the psychosocial-psychodynamic model this wasn't necessarily considered to be long stay.

One patient who had been there over a year was Mr. L., the eldest son of the military dictator of a small African country. As the eldest son, he had been groomed to be his father's successor. He had developed schizoaffective disorder in his early twenties and was instead consigned to hospital.

He was now in his early thirties, and a large man both in frame and in weight—very strong and sometimes violent. On one occasion, he was placed in four-point mechanical restraint after one of his violent episodes (meaning that he was secured to his bed by padded cuffs on arms and legs,) yet he was strong enough to somehow rock the bed about sufficiently that, when we heard noises coming from the restraint room and went down to check, we found him walking about with the bed strapped on his back, like a turtle. (This was in the days when a patient in restraints was not routinely on constant staff observation.)

He was very proud of his strength, often loudly proclaiming: "I have balls… like bull!"

The procedure at the hospital was that the staff member doing safety checks on patients would also have the duty of opening the unit door to let patients on and off the unit, providing they had the ordered privileges to do so.

One day I had this duty for the usual hour, during which Mr. L. asked me to open the door for him. I checked his privilege status in the nursing station and found that he was restricted to the unit at that time. When I told him this, he initially started his familiar outraged blustering, but when he figured that this wasn't going to work, he calmed down and said that he had an offer to make me.

I expected him to say something along the usual lines of giving me money if I opened the door or a threat if I didn't, but instead he looked me steadily in the eye and said, "If you open the door for me, I will make you Emperor of the Universe."

I was charmed by his offer, and for the glimpse it gave me into true grandiose thinking. For he was perfectly serious when he made it, and to be able to make another person Emperor of the Universe meant that he himself had power way beyond that role. I told him that I very much appreciated his generous offer, but that I liked working at the hospital and just didn't want to get fired.

Thought: grandiosity is certainly a feature of some affective disorders, and in this case, was reinforced by the grandiosity engendered by Mr. L.'s highly privileged upbringing. His wonderful offer to me helped me appreciate how difficult it must be for patients with grandiose thinking to bear what to them are mere petty rules enforced by inferior underlings.

I hadn't been involved in using mechanical restraints until I worked in US hospitals, and I was initially quite shocked to see a patient in four-point restraint. The reason mechanical restraint was used almost routinely in the US, while not at all in the UK is an interesting question. Part of the answer is probably that, in that era, British society generally was simply not so violent as American society, and this was reflected in the psychiatric population, where I could readily see that violent behavior was much less common in the UK than in the US. (See Sketch # 80.) I don't know if that still holds true now, but it did in the era that I lived and worked in the UK.

The other part of the picture is that, while I never saw mechanical restraint used in UK psychiatric hospitals, this was in some degree due to smoke and mirrors in how dangerous clinical situations were handled. For violent behavior that would have automatically resulted in four-point restraint in the US did indeed occur in the UK, even if far less often, and when it did, it usually resulted in the patient receiving restraint through chemical injection, and being physically held by staff for as long as it took to have the medication calm the patient down (see Sketch #28.)

In the end, handling violent patient behavior with physical and chemical restraint is probably actually very little different from using mechanical restraint.

Sketch # 39

A patient called Mr. L. had a beat-up old Thunderbird car that he kept on grounds and drove around the area for an hour whenever he had the privilege to do so. Driving his car appeared to mean more to him than anything else in the world, and the possibility of being able to use it was the one thing that staff members could use to prompt him to behave safely over a period of time.

One day I asked him why driving the car was so important to him. His reply was, "Here on the unit I'm told what to do every minute of my life by you people. I'm told when to get up, when to take medications, when to eat, what groups to go to. But when I'm in my car, I make the decisions! I decide where to go and what roads to use to get there. I decide whether to turn right or turn left or to drive straight on. I am in control, not you!"

Thought: Control is an issue in everyone's life, and it is a big issue on psychiatric units. Staff members must ultimately be in control if the unit is to remain safe, but if they become too dogmatic and controlling over every minor issue, then in the end the unit becomes unsafe. Psychiatric staff members should look for little ways in which patients can make decisions for themselves, for that will be meaningful to them and make them more inclined to work with the treatment team on the big issues.

Sketch # 40

When I had worked in psychiatry in England in the 1970s there were certainly patients with substance abuse diagnoses (usually alcoholism), but it was unusual to find a patient with dual psychiatric and substance abuse diagnoses. But when I starting to work in the United States in the early 1980s, I noticed that such dual diagnosis patients were not unusual at all, and over the next thirty years, they were to become almost the norm.

One such person was a young man in his late twenties who had the psychiatric diagnosis of paranoid schizophrenia and the additional diagnosis of polysubstance abuse.

He had periodic auditory hallucinations that warned him of threats to his life. When sober, he rarely responded to these voices, but when he was taking alcohol or any street drug that he could obtain, he became more volatile and agitated. His belief, however, was that the drugs helped him to deal with the anxiety that he always felt due to these threats against him.

On the unit, he often tried to persuade other patients who had privileges to go off the hospital grounds to buy drugs for him and smuggle them back onto the unit. When nothing else was forthcoming, he would suck the alcoholic liquid out of magic markers given to other patients to make pictures or posters with. He would sometimes appear at the nursing station with green or some other colored ink all around his mouth, having just sucked on a pen, and with a straight face ask staff members if he could now have another color as he needed to finish his picture. He would then be shocked and outraged when they refused.

Every now and then he would try to rush out of the door when it was being opened for another patient. Even when he was occasionally successful in this, there was generally not the rapid response mobilization by staff that there would certainly be if another patient had escaped. Instead, a staff member would simply call the hospital's campus police, who would then wait for a few minutes before leisurely driving up to the liquor store half a mile away from the hospital. Almost without fail they would find him there either trying to buy or shoplift some beer, and would then bring him back to the unit, and he always returned without any struggle. The liquor store staff themselves even started to call the campus police when the patient came in, as they knew what was happening.

Thought: Dual-diagnosis patients have probably become the most difficult of all patients to treat because they often refuse to take psychiatric medications while insisting that street drugs are helpful to them. This group of patients may engage in criminal activities in order to satisfy their drug cravings, and consequently end up in jails rather than hospitals, with their mental status often then deteriorating. Poor judgement leads to inadvertent overdosing, with heroin-related deaths particularly a current deadly epidemic in the United States. These days it is basically impossible to effectively run a psychiatric program of any description if it doesn't include some substance abuse components.

Sketch # 41

This sketch of an incident at the hospital did not involve me personally, but it was a meaningful one, so I will relate it.

On the psycho-geriatric unit one day, a nurse went to a room to talk to a patient. There she found the patient actively cutting his wrists with some glass from a broken bottle. She yelled for help and then instinctively ran toward him and tried to grab his arm to stop him from cutting himself.

The patient then turned to her and stabbed her in the left eye with the glass.

The patient lived, but the nurse was permanently blinded in that eye.

Thoughts: A lot of people have thoughts of killing themselves at times, but it takes a particularly intense mental state to actually attempt to do it. When people get themselves into a state in which their single focus is on actively killing themselves, then even if they have to kill someone else in order to achieve that goal, they will do that.

Psychiatric nurses must therefore be very conscious of the risks if they intervene alone in an active suicide attempt, especially one in which a weapon is involved. In the end, we will do what our conscience tells us to do, but nurses should always call for help before putting their own safety in jeopardy.

At the time of this incident, a staff member going into a patient room alone was routine, and not in itself any particular danger (See Sketch # 24). But as the general acuity of psychiatric inpatient units has increased over the years, and insurance companies have started to refuse to pay acute inpatient rates for less-acute patients, this apparently simple action has become more problematic for staff.

Certainly, nurses working on a forensic psychiatric unit should never go into a patient room by themselves. At a later time, I worked in a forensic psychiatric hospital in which a patient, in his room at the most distant end of the unit, requested to see a nurse, saying that he was feeling sick. The unit staff members were all otherwise occupied that this time, so one of the nurses went by herself to see what was wrong with him. The patient then came very close to successfully raping her in the shower before his roommate alerted staff to what was going on.

In principle, on any inpatient psychiatric unit these days, nurses should never put themselves out of the line of sight of another staff member. At the very least, if it's one of those hectic times on a unit when another staff member simply can't be found to help, a nurse should always tell at least one other staff member that he or she intends to go into a patient room. At least that way, someone will be able to keep some sort of track of the nurse.

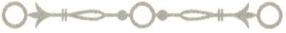

The hospital at this time was a leader in diagnosing and treating patients with borderline personality disorder. I had never even heard of the diagnosis when I worked in England.

Borderline personality disordered (BPD) patients are never easy for staff to treat, due to their impulsivity and ability to instantly distort and misinterpret reality. So, if we were told that our next admission to the unit had that diagnosis, there would often be a collective groan from staff. One of the veteran mental health workers on the unit, M. M. would refer to the intense, dramatic behaviors often seen with BPD patients as "wicked bodo action," and this phrase became part of the staff's regular language when behind closed doors.

It was part of the diagnosis and treatment process at this hospital to have a psychiatrist expert in that diagnosis come to the unit after a while to personally interview the patient, have the case presented to him or her by the treatment team, and then make treatment recommendations. And so, with newly admitted "borderline" patients, a consultation with the expert psychiatrist would be arranged. Staff members would often dread this consultation as the usually assigned expert psychiatrist, Dr. G. J., was very direct in his interviews with patients, and it was commonplace for them to become either self-mutilatory or assaultive a short while after the interview concluded, not infrequently requiring mechanical restraint.

Sketch # 42

Ms. L. was in her late thirties and worked as a licensed practical nurse at a nursing home a few miles from the hospital. She'd had a series of admissions to the unit for self-mutilatory behaviors (usually cutting her forearms) associated with borderline personality disorder. On the unit, she would continue to have periods of scratching herself, or banging her head on the wall, that could become so protracted or severe that she had to be placed in four-point restraint to stop her from doing serious injury to herself.

One morning we came onto the unit at the start of the first shift to find her in restraints because she had assaulted a staff member an hour earlier. Even when an inpatient herself, she wanted to go to her regular job as often as possible, as she was afraid that she would be fired otherwise, and the job had an important role in maintaining her fragile stability.

While this would be usually impossible with patients in other diagnostic categories, it was occasionally possible with BPD patients to do this due to the ability of some to psychologically recompensate just as quickly as they could decompensate.

We went to assess her in restraints after shift report. We found her calm, and she asked if she could be released to go to work. She gave assurances about her safety, and presented as oriented and stable, so we released her. She had a quick shower and then drove off in her car to go to receive her own nursing shift report at the nursing home!

Our hearts were in our mouths when she left, as even good assessments are not guarantees, so we were very relieved when she called the unit back from the nursing home's telephone as we had asked her to do.

She returned to the unit at the end of her shift, reporting that she had an enjoyable day.

On another occasion, our assessment of her status was not so good. She had been allowed to leave the unit to go to work, and when driving she noticed a police car a couple of cars behind her. She immediately started to have paranoid ideas about whether the police could be following her specifically, and why this might be happening. Ending up being fearful for her life, she therefore accelerated toward the nursing home with the police then in hot pursuit. The high-speed chase ended with her pulling up in front of the facility and running inside to her unit in the apparent belief that this would offer her sanctuary from the police.

The incident ended with the police returning her to the hospital without pressing charges. At that point, she did not go back to her regular nursing job until she had been discharged from our unit.

Thoughts: BPD patients are often dreaded by staff as they frequently behave in various provocative, unsafe ways. The inevitable cycle then becomes that the more unsafely the patient behaves, the more staff members feel compelled to respond in ever-more controlling ways to ensure safety, with the patient then figuring out ever-more inventive ways to circumvent these safety measures and to harm themselves. Treatment then, in effect, grinds to a halt, with both the patient and the staff feeling frustrated and angry.

Patients can't break this cycle as that's their illness, so it is up to the treatment team and staff members to break it. As Ms. L. demonstrated when she went directly from four-point restraints to her regular job, staff members being willing to take seemingly paradoxical steps that would probably never be considered with other patients may work with this group of patients.

In all branches of nursing, sometimes the intensity and emotionally draining nature of the work can lead staff to adopting a "black humor" regarding some patients. Unit staff referring here to the unsafe behaviors of a BPD patient as "wicked bodo action" would be an example of this. This is a normal and healthy way of dealing with the stresses of the job, as long as it stays behind closed doors, between staff members, but it should never be used in front of patients, as this would certainly be seen as staff being demeaning toward them, which would make a treatment alliance with them all the more difficult.

Working with patients with the diagnosis of borderline personality as well as other personality disorders will, from time to time, present nurses with a well-known trap: the patient will say to the nurse something like, "I like you and I trust you. There's something I need to tell you, but I can't tell you unless you promise not to tell anyone else. Will you promise not to tell?"

Unwary nurses can be flattered by what the patient has said, and in then believing that they must be a superior clinician to their peers, may be tempted into agreeing not to share what the patient says to them. This is a trap, though, because on the one hand if the nurse promises not to tell anyone else, and the patient then tells him, for instance, that she has a plan to kill herself that afternoon, then the nurse would, of course, have to instantly break his or her promise and alert everyone else of the danger. And, on the other hand, if the nurse agrees not to tell anyone else, and what the patient says is something that the nurse believes isn't important enough to inform the treatment team about, then the nurse has now entered into a secret, personal, unprofessional relationship with the patient, one that will very probably end badly. For the patient will then start to manipulate the nurse into doing things that the nurse knows are not appropriate, and if the nurse refuses to do those things, the patient will quickly inform the rest of the treatment team about their secret arrangement, and the nurse will be left to explain and defend dangerously unprofessional conduct.

When patients tell nurses that they have something important to tell them, but will only do so if they promise to tell no one else, the standard reply must be similar to this: "I would very much like to hear what you have to say, but if it's anything that would affect your care and treatment here, then I am professionally obliged to share that with your treatment team. Please tell me what you have to say, so that I can make sure that the treatment team can give you the best care possible."

Most often, when nurses say this and patients know that the nurses will pass on what they say, they will then tell the nurses what they were going to say anyway. (See Sketch # 24.)

Sketch # 43

Ms. Y. was a twenty-five-year-old woman admitted with agitation, anxiety, and confusion. She spoke very quickly, her concentration was poor, and she would quickly forget people's names. With a prior history of bipolar disorder, she was provisionally diagnosed as being in a hypomanic state and was started on the common treatment combination of haloperidol and lithium carbonate.

Several days after her admission, Ms. Y. experienced some muscle rigidity. It was of a constant unyielding nature, unlike the "cogwheel" rigidity seen in Parkinsonian reactions. Her confusion became worse, and at times she became mute. She developed tachycardia (a rapid heart rate caused by a problem in the heart's electrical system) and a low-grade fever with swinging blood pressure also noted a day later.

Due to her confused state, her ability to maintain her own safety on a locked unit was evident, so she was nursed in a single room on five-minute safety checks while her medications were discontinued due to the possibility of part of her clinical presentation being due to side effects of those medications.

Over the next six days, Ms. Y. at times appeared alert, but was also often dazed and almost stuporous, and was therefore placed on one-on-one staff observation. She started to sweat profusely, and it took considerable staff persistence to maintain a satisfactory fluid intake with her. Several neurological examinations took place on the unit, but findings were inconclusive.

Finally, after another four days, she was transferred to a local general hospital where elevated creatinine phosphokinase levels were noted, and she was given a diagnosis of neuroleptic malignant syndrome (NMS), a potentially fatal side effect of some antipsychotic medications. She eventually recovered.

The reaction of other patients on the unit to this developing scenario was initially (and rather surprisingly to me) one of anger toward Ms. Y. Some patients even verbally abused her personally and demanded that she be transferred off the unit. They appeared to see her as a competitor for staff time and attention because, with her being initially checked every five minutes and then on one-on-one monitoring, there was less time for staff to pay attention to them.

This was particularly true of the patients with personality disorders, two of whom started to express increasingly urgent suicidal and self-mutilatory ideas as Ms. Y.'s condition deteriorated, requiring them also to be placed on increased staff observation as she had been.

On the other hand, patients with the diagnosis of schizophrenia appeared to actually clinically improve in the face of Ms. Y's clearly serious illness. This may have actually been due to staff not being able to spend as much time with them as usual, as people with schizophrenia most often feel more comfortable when they have less contact with other people. It has been the observation of many psychiatric nurses that, when patients with schizophrenia become physically ill themselves, their psychosis may clear up somewhat, and possibly that same phenomenon was at work here, even with the sick person being another person.

When it was finally established that Ms. Y.'s illness was actually an iatrogenic illness (illness caused by the treatment itself), patients' anger toward her became anger toward staff members. Several patients even demanded that they be allowed to leave the hospital, and others refused to take their medications. Only the existence of long-standing, solid staff-patient relationships along with intensive personal and group education on the use of medications eventually re-established patient trust in their treaters and treatment, preventing what could have developed into chaos on the unit.

Staff reaction to this scenario was initially one of frustration as they looked on apparently helplessly as Ms. Y.'s illness relentlessly deteriorated. Above all, nurses want to help sick people, but here we appeared to be unable to help her in any way, conflicting with the role-image that we had of ourselves. The feelings of frustration and helplessness among the nurses then turned into anger toward the unit administrators who expected them care effectively for a patient when the nurses felt the care required skills that they did not necessarily have. For, just as many general nurses don't feel at all comfortable caring for psychiatric patients on medical and surgical units, so many psychiatric nurses feel that they have lost many of the skills required to safely care for medically sick patients.

Staff members then demanded that the patient be discharged to a general hospital. Their anger became mixed with guilt once it became probably that Ms. Y.'s illness was an iatrogenic one, and that further mixed with fear that there might be a lawsuit should the patient die as a result of her illness. The situation on the unit remained tense until she actually was transferred.

Thought: Looking back on it, I find it is odd that it took so long before this patient's medical condition was accurately identified, and we were perhaps lucky that the patient fully recovered from it. At that time, NMS was simply not on our radar to the degree that it rightfully is now, as deaths from it can be as high as 20 percent.

Much has been written about the problems of having an actively psychiatrically ill patient in a general hospital setting, but less about the problems of having an actively medically ill patient in a psychiatric setting. But in both cases, patients can unwittingly become seriously disruptive to the care being provided to others on their ward or unit, and nurses should be alert to any problems that develop.

When an iatrogenic patient injury or illness occurs, nurses must quickly respond to the inevitable legitimate anxieties of other patients about their own treatment, whether they are vocalized or not. In this case, staff members held many group and individual sessions devoted entirely to exploring such patient anxieties and reassuring them where possible. Several copies of the *Physicians' Desk Reference* (PDR) were left in patient areas in an effort to demonstrate that we were being transparent and honest in their treatment, and nurses were available to answer whatever questions they had. Many of the questions and complaints that patients had about their medications were familiar ones, as patients often do not like to take them anyway, but just having staff not avoiding their concerns was a reassurance in itself.

Though the temptation to become defensive may be strong when the fear of a lawsuit is in the back of staff members' minds, that fear must be addressed only in staff meetings with management and the whole treatment team. Becoming defensive on legal issues directly with patients only leads to their quickly identifying staff members' defensiveness as such, causing them to worry that they are therefore not safe on the unit

Sketch # 44

Nursing stations are the Times Squares of inpatient psychiatric units; there's usually a lot of action going on there.

Patients will be up there asking for anything from toothpaste to discharge papers, demanding a room change, asking when their psychiatrist is due in, or if their attorney is coming that day. On and on it goes. Hypomanic patients will be talking excitedly to any staff member or patient who will listen to them, while sociopathic patients will be either angrily complaining about their rights being violated or amiably chatting with staff, looking to gain some insights into their personal lives just in case they may need their cooperation at some later time. Paranoid patients will be quietly gliding around a few yards away avoiding direct contact with staff but hoping to glean some clues as to what plots are being hatched against them, while psychotic patients will be sitting in corridor chairs staring intently at staff at the nursing station, trying to figure out who these creatures are who have so much power over their lives.

Sometimes a patient becomes so angry at not getting the answers they want that they try to jump into the nursing station to assault staff. And sometimes they succeed.

Thoughts: Being at the unit nursing station dealing with dozens of patient issues is often an exhausting assignment, and the temptation can be to lighten the load by bantering with each other about personal or work issues. But nurses are paid to treat the patients, and their personal goal must be to provide professional care to them, so this is a temptation to be avoided.

Nurses should carefully avoid complaining in front of patients about their colleagues on other shifts not doing their jobs properly. They must not complain about their managers, psychiatrists, staffing levels, or general hospital issues in front of patients. Those are issues that should be discussed in staff areas behind closed doors. Once patients see that staff members are more absorbed by their own issues rather than in caring for them, then effective treatment becomes much more difficult.

Similarly, nurses must be very careful not to talk about their personal lives with patients, no matter how natural it may seem at a given moment. For delusional patients may well end up incorporating these details and their nurses into their delusional systems, while personality disordered patients may use them to try to compromise the nurse if it ever suits them to do so. If a nurse tells a patient where he or she buys groceries, the nurse shouldn't be shocked to meet the patient there at some point in the future.

And even if there are no patients actually standing at the nursing station, nurses should try to avoid talking about personal issues with colleagues in such patient areas, as it's an easy habit to get into but a far less easy one to break.

Sketch # 45

As all nurses know, the first and second shifts are entirely different creatures. On the first shift, there are frequent individual meetings with doctors, psychologists, social workers, and others. There are treatment team meetings, meetings with the unit manager, and more. The number of such meetings may leave little time for anything else, including meaningful interactions with patients.

But on the second shift, most of the other treatment team members and the manager have gone home. The shift supervisor will swing by briefly to ask if everything is okay, but otherwise the staff nurse is left alone to be his or her own master or mistress. There will be lots of time to interact with patients if he or she wants to. And a lot of nurses choose to work that shift for those very reasons.

I liked that shift and liked being on the unit with patients, then going back to the conference room to talk with the other staff members about what was happening on the unit. As time went on, I found that other staff members were gradually asking me more and more to discuss their assigned patients with them, so I found that I was spending more time in the conference room and less on the unit.

Almost without really noticing it myself, I became less of a staff nurse working directly with patients, and more of a charge nurse working with staff on how best to provide care to their patients. And I slowly found myself enjoying talking with staff on how best to handle clinical situations that were developing on the unit.

After about a year, a shift supervisor position in the hospital's central nursing office became vacant, and some staff members suggested that I should apply for it. My first reaction was negative, largely because I had been active in health unions from the very beginning and being in management just didn't seem to fit in with how I saw myself.

But it did make sense to me from one point of view: for some time on the unit, I had been largely clinically supervising staff rather than directly providing care myself, and I had found that this was actually an effective way of keeping the unit reasonably stable and providing good patient care. So I did wonder, if I was able to have a role on the unit that helped patients get good care, perhaps I would also be able to fill a role that could similarly help patients throughout the hospital.

Like every other nurse, I was very aware that individual supervisors could make significant differences on how easy or how difficult it could be for staff members to effectively run their units, and I wondered if I had the ability to make it easier for them.

So I applied for the position, and I got it. And for the next twenty-five years, to my often-bemused surprise, I found myself working in middle, and then executive, nursing management positions.

Thought: I have seen some ambitious nurses carefully and successfully plan out every detail of their career in advance. But the rest of us should simply be aware of any changes that may be taking place in ourselves and in our professional priorities, and carefully consider opportunities as they come up even if at first glimpse we would consider them to be not what we are looking for.

Sketch # 46

England is a small country, broken up geographically into very small counties. There are no differences among the counties regarding the legal aspects of mental health; all of that is determined by national UK laws.

America is a very large country broken up into large states, each of which has a certain amount of legal autonomy, including laws relating to mental health.

I didn't understand this important difference when I became a shift supervisor at this hospital, but I soon learned.

A patient escaped one day, and nothing was heard of her for several days. I was working on the day shift the following weekend when a halfway house in Maine called us on Sunday to say that she had turned up there. I therefore had a Massachusetts "pink paper" completed, legally authorizing her return to the hospital. I had seen this done several times before and assumed that I could do it on this case also. I sent three mental health workers in a car up to Maine to bring her back using the authority of that document, which they did without any difficulties.

I had Monday off, and when I came back to work on Tuesday, there was uproar over what I had done. To my shock, I learned from the hospital legal department that what I had done in transporting a patient across state lines on the sole authority of a Massachusetts document legally constituted kidnapping, and that both the hospital and I could be successfully sued as a result.

Fortunately, no such suits followed, but I was very quickly brought up to speed regarding "state's rights" in the United States!

Thought: whenever legal documents are concerned, when doing something for the first time, even if they are perfectly confident that what they are doing is right, nurses should run their intentions by someone else (preferably their supervisors) before doing it!

Sketch # 47

Shift supervisors soon learn the value of a calm, competent staff nurse. There'll be days when a unit nurse will call the staffing office begging for and demanding extra staff "because the place is nearly out of control!" So the shift supervisor will look for a unit that appears to be reasonably quiet and send a staff member from there to help out on the busy unit.

Then, when the supervisor does rounds on the quiet, minus-one-staff-member unit, the nurse will say, "That unit's always chaotic because they have no idea what they're doing. We keep our unit quiet and in control, so why are we being punished for doing our job properly by having to run understaffed just to help a unit that isn't doing a proper job?"

At first, I would take that complaint with a pinch of salt, but over time, I found that there was often a lot of truth in it. For the units who often called the staffing office at the start of the shift requesting more staff were the same units that always seemed to be having clinical crises, were always complaining about taking a new admission, and always opposed to sending one of their staff members to help another unit even for a short time.

Sometimes populations that consisted of the more difficult patients played a part in the seemingly permanently chaos in those units, but almost always a major factor was that the staff nurses didn't know how to supervise their direct care staff properly, and didn't have good milieu management skills or the ability to effectively resolve clinical situations on the unit.

And almost always, the managers of these units, instead of working with their nurses to improve their supervisory and clinical skills, would buy into the staff members' complaints that the only problem on the unit was that they weren't being given enough staff.

These unit managers would therefore often come to the staffing office with the same list of allegedly unreasonable expectations being placed upon their unit, always ending with demands for more staff to meet these expectations. These units all had the same culture of viewing themselves as being victims of "the system." The staff members of all disciplines were never happy, and the units were rarely clinically stable or productive.

On the other hand, managers who didn't instantly buy into their staff members' complaints without looking first into seeing if they were justified or not invariably supervised settled staff and ran clinically settled units.

So I started to see that it wasn't so much the quality of the staff nurses alone that determined how well a unit ran; over time, it became clear to me that the unit manager's role was the really crucial one in having a professional, well-run, and clinically effective unit. And, inevitably, I wondered how I would do in that role.

So, after two years in the staffing office, I applied for an open manager position and started work on a small unit serving patients with psychotic illnesses, with the treatment based on biological psychiatry principles.

Thoughts: As a staff nurse on a constantly busy unit, it's often tempting to take the easy way out regarding the volume of work on the unit and the staffing available. Managers who experience a good shift or enjoy a stable period value it and don't want it to end. On several shifts when I was the unit charge nurse, I was asked to take an admission but falsely claimed that we were far too busy to take one, even though we were actually enjoying a perfectly good shift and had an empty bed. And direct-care staff will almost always encourage their nurses to take that easy way out, and praise them when they do, as it usually means less work for them. And it can become tempting for nurses to place a priority on pleasing the direct care-staff and becoming popular with them.

If that mind-set becomes permanent, then the professional culture on the unit does deteriorate, and it's the job of the unit manager to make sure that doesn't happen. It's his or her job to support, encourage, teach, and sometimes set limits on the nurses so that they can become confident professionals able to handle the weird and wonderful things that will inevitably confront them, rather than becoming chronic complainers on chronically chaotic units.

Sketch # 48

As a new unit manager, I had the responsibility of hiring new unit staff. The first person I interviewed was an applicant for a mental health worker position. He had good credentials, experience, and ambitions, but I found myself just not liking him. He seemed smug somehow. But I asked the personnel department staff to offer him the job, as on paper he seemed theoretically like a perfectly good candidate.

I later talked about this with T. K., the unit manager who had been assigned as my mentor during my manager orientation. She was a veteran manager who had seen it all. She was smart and pithy, a great person to have as a mentor. She told me this: "Never hire someone you find yourself not liking, as he or she will just end up being a torment to you. There are plenty of people with good resumes and plenty of people who can give the right answers in an interview. But If you find yourself not even enjoying talking to them, even if you don't understand why, never hire them to work for you."

Over the years, I found that this was very sensible advice. People can certainly work well with peers or superiors whom they may not personally like, but when it comes to supervising people, it is very helpful to have a positive feeling about them.

In this case I was fortunate, as the candidate refused the job offer.

Another thing that my mentor told me that turned out to be very true was this: "One of the main roles of managers, whether they're in middle management or executive management, is to protect those staff members below them from the craziness of those above them!" And, indeed, in both middle and executive management positions, I did find that a lot of my time and energy as a manager was spent in ameliorating the worst effects of some of the policy decisions of those above me.

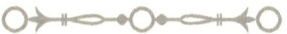

Shortly before I started working as a unit manager, one of the RNs there said that she was going to transfer to another unit. She had enjoyed working with the previous manager so much that she didn't believe that a similar situation could be replicated with a new one.

I knew from my time in the staffing office that this nurse was an unusually good one, and I was anxious about her leaving, believing that the unit would not run so well without her. I talked to my mentor about my concerns, to which she replied: "Don't worry about things that you can't control. She is a good nurse, and you can certainly talk to her about what might be concerning her, but if she wants to go, then she goes. In management, the coming and going of staff will be a never-ending constant in your life, and you have to roll with it."

And she was right: good nurses come, and good nurses sometimes go even if managers try hard to keep them. Managers can't totally stop worrying about this, but they also can't exhaust all of their mental energy trying to stop a process that can't be stopped.

Thought: People who are in a position to assign a mentor to a person in a new role should choose someone who is experienced and has had personal knowledge of what he or she is talking about, rather than, for instance, a person recently out of graduate school who may just end up relating advice learned during a lecture as he or she simply hasn't had time to actually gain personal experience.

Sketch # 49

When I became a unit manager, I had my own office for the first time. I then started to wonder what I should put on the walls of my office, figuring that sometimes people who came to meet with me might look around the room either to find a conversation piece or to gain some insights into what I might value.

Some people put up their framed academic qualifications, and some people put up inspirational sayings or beautiful landscapes. I have an interest in history, so as my first office hanging, I bought a nice Florence Nightingale signature clipped from one of her letters, and had it framed with some pictures from her time in the Crimean War. I thought that this would be a good talking point if someone was looking for one.

As time went by, I added other pictures, usually posters about nursing or photographs of hospitals.

Contrary to what I expected, over the course of the next twenty-plus years of having my own offices, with the single exception of a psychiatrist who liked an architect's draft drawing of an old asylum, not a single person ever commented on any of the pictures in them. Not a single nurse ever appeared to notice the Nightingale autograph.

Thought: New managers obsessing about how best to set up their offices shouldn't worry too much about what pictures to put up. As it turns out, people come into these offices, talk with the managers, and leave. They may cast their eyes about the room, but they're probably not actually taking much in; they're just organizing their thoughts.

Maybe other managers have had different experiences, and maybe I just didn't have interesting enough stuff, but based on my experience, my advice on this issue would be: put up pictures that bring personal enjoyment; no one else will most likely look at them!

Sketch # 50

At the time that I became a unit manager, my wife was also a manager of an inpatient unit at the hospital. This was an unusual situation, one that caused some consternation in some other members of the nursing management group who had the fear that my wife and I would form a subgroup within the larger group, always supporting each other's positions simply because we were married rather than on the merits of any issue.

At the hospital in that era, clinical boundaries between staff and patients was a focus of care, correctly recognizing the dangers that boundary violations present to effective treatment. But that focus appeared to give the nursing department the confidence that they could, therefore, handle what might appear at first sight to be a potentially problematic boundary issue. Simply, they had the confidence to do what other hospitals might shy away from.

So my wife and I attended all of the same meetings and even sat on the same committees.

And there were no real problems, probably because we were both supervised by the assistant director of nursing, T. D., a smart and subtle manager who had good antennae for any developing problems.

Thought: This was a parallel situation to the one frequently encountered amongst unit staff—it is usually a hospital policy that close family members cannot work together on the same shift on the same unit.

The logic of this is that these family ties may override clinical or ethical considerations when it comes to making decisions on how to best handle a particular patient situation, or in responding to allegations of patient abuse or otherwise breaking hospital and departmental policies.

Putting a good nurse in the situation where he or she has to make the choice between saying that his or her family member abused a patient and should be fired or saying that he or she "saw and heard nothing" is one that a hospital should obviously avoid for everyone's sake.

Sketch # 51

There was an emergency admission to the unit one afternoon—a man in his early forties who had a long history of paranoid schizophrenia. He had been living in a halfway house for some time but had recently been refusing his medications and had started to become suspicious of and defiant to staff members to the point that he could no longer be safely treated in that setting.

He came directly onto the unit rather than through the admissions office. He was surrounded by staff and campus police, his clothes were dirty and rumpled, and he looked very frightened. The unit protocol was to search direct admissions for weapons or other contraband in the "quiet room," so he was taken there.

He went in, but when he was asked to take his overcoat off, he became very agitated, started yelling that the staff were taking him into the room with the intention of torturing and raping him, then killing him. He charged out of the room screaming, and a physical restraint followed.

The best description that I ever heard of the physical restraint process is "organized chaos." And that's exactly what it is. For no matter how well trained the staff members are, when they are actually trying to safely immobilize a large man who truly believes that he is fighting for his life, many things can go wrong. Staff members who are assigned to hold a particular limb may lose their grip, a staff member may lose his or her balance and fall down. Any number of things can happen; the process just never goes as easily in real life as it does in training.

And while this physical restraint was certainly organized chaos, it still appeared to be a normal restraint, heading inevitably toward the usual ending. After about two minutes, the patient was no longer struggling, and staff members were starting to lift him up to take him back to the quiet room to be placed in four-point restraint.

At that point, the staff member directing the restraint yelled that the patient did not appear to be breathing. A medical emergency code was called. CPR was done, and the EMTs came, but the patient was dead.

We were all stunned. In our worst nightmares, we had never thought that this would ever happen, as everyone was very well trained and experienced in real-life restraints. Yet now it had happened; our patient was dead.

We were starting to try to figure it all out when a new nurse quietly said: "I heard him say, 'I can't breathe.'" No one else had heard it, but the patient had said it, and one person had heard it.

We remained stunned for a long time. We had prided ourselves that we could safely handle the most clinically acute situations, but now a patient in our care had died.

Months of detailed legal, administrative, and clinical reviews followed and were concluded, but every one of us there remembers that terrible day very clearly. At the time, some individuals told me that the best resolution to the whole tragedy would be for me to identify the mental health worker in charge of the restraint as being negligent in his duties and fire him or her. But I couldn't see how that person was negligent, and it seemed wrong to unfairly pick out a scapegoat for the tragedy just to do it. The hospital administration never put on any pressure on me to do this, even though it may have made the situation legally simpler for them, and I appreciated that. It made me realize what a truly professionally run hospital it was.

Thoughts: psychiatric nursing, like all branches of nursing, can involve life-and-death issues. Usually in psychiatry we think of that applying to suicide, but every nurse should be aware that it can also apply to the restraint process.

When nurses are working with clinically acute, agitated patients, there are many times when there is ultimately no safe option but to restrain the patient. But, as I found out to my horror, even with good, well-trained staff, in the chaos that a restraint inevitably involves there is always the potential for something terrible to happen.

So patients should be restrained only as a last resort, and the restraint should be conducted as a potential life-and-death process.

Additionally, and importantly, nurses who hear or see something unsafe going on in *any* clinical process, should yell it out to everyone else. Even novice psychiatric nurses who feel that everyone else must know better what is happening and what to do must have the confidence to make sure that everyone is aware of what they are aware of.

Patient deaths during restraints has rightly become a national topic of discussion over the past decade, yet there remains no national consensus on what is the safest way to restrain a patient.

For instance, in Massachusetts, we always had to place patients in four-point restraint so that they were lying on their stomachs, on the basis that the most pressing danger to patients in restraints was that they might

Wonderful and Weird

vomit, and if they were restrained on their backs, they could then choke on that vomit.

On the other hand, when I worked in Ohio, it was a firing offense to restrain patients on their stomachs on the basis that the most pressing danger to a patient in restraints was that they might be unable to breathe freely, and that restraining them on their backs was the safest way of ensuring that they could do this.

It would surely be very helpful for patient safety if there could be some definitive national clinical consensus on how best to restrain a patient.

Sketch # 52

At a teaching hospital, there are opportunities to go to interesting clinical conferences, and I went to as many as I could.

At one of these, the main speaker, who was not a nurse, started his presentation by saying this: "Nursing is unique as a profession in that it has as its founder and inspirational figure, a prostitute."

He was referring to Florence Nightingale. I was astonished at his statement, as this was the first time I had ever heard this, though I have heard several people say it since. Simply, it's a lie that is told by people who have never taken the trouble to study Nightingale's life.

When I told the speaker that what he had said was simply not true, he apologized, saying that he was only repeating what he had been told. But he gave me the distinct impression that the next time he gave that same talk, he would start off making the same statement.

I was interested that the audience was made up entirely of nurses, yet no one else challenged the speaker's statement that Nightingale was a prostitute.

Thought: The idea that Florence Nightingale was a prostitute is a lie, yet it persists. I think that this is because nursing, a female-dominated profession, is not infrequently the subject of sexual fantasies by men outside of nursing, a fantasy actively encouraged by the pornography industry. Physical nursing care and "sexual healing" are not always concepts carefully differentiated when it comes to male sexual fantasies.

When I worked in general hospitals in England, black pantyhose was an essential part of the nurse's uniform. In many ways, this could certainly be legitimately viewed as simply a centuries-long tradition, but at the same time, of all of the potential colors for pantyhose, black also culturally carried with it the most sexually suggestive overtones.

When male patients were being discharged, it was common for them to give small gifts to the nurses in appreciation for the care given to them. Often this would be a box of chocolates, but not infrequently it would be a pair of these black tights. If you asked patients why they were giving nurses pantyhose, they would say it was simply to save the nurse the expense of buying them themselves and would be genuinely horrified at the thought that there was any sexual motive in giving that particular gift (11).

But at the unconscious level, a man giving black underwear as a gift to a young woman cannot fail to bring with it some sexual meaning. And it is this fantasy level thinking that reveals itself openly when speakers refer to Nightingale as being a prostitute.

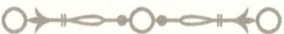

While gift giving by grateful patients to nurses is common in general nursing, psychiatric nurses soon find out that it's different in their chosen field.

A psychiatric patient offering a nurse a gift is actually so unusual that, when it does happen, the nurse must always discuss it with his or her supervisor, to try to figure out if there is some hidden agenda to why the gift was offered. For instance, is the patient becoming sexually attracted to the nurse? Will the acceptance of the gift then be viewed as encouraging pursuit? A sociopathic patient may be offering a gift in order to make the nurse feel obliged to him or her in some way. A few days later the patient could ask the nurse to do something, such as smuggling in cigarettes or drugs.

In general, the best route for a nurse to take when offered a gift by a patient is to say something like: "I appreciate your kind thought, but there are hospital rules against my accepting the gift." (There will be such a policy.) The nurse should then tell his or her supervisor and colleagues.

I think that the reason psychiatric patients rarely offer nurses gifts is related to the widespread phenomenon of patients denying their mental illnesses. For when patients do not believe that they are ill in the first place, they don't believe that they need to be in hospital, or take medications. To them, the ministrations of nurses may well be more annoying than appreciated.

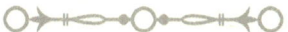

Nurses should always attend any interesting conference that they have an opportunity to go to, as they never know if they'll have the same opportunities in their next job!

Sketch # 53

In the late 1980s, the nursing department decided to establish the "Marker Model" as the practice model for its nurses to follow at the hospital (12).

Carolyn Marker came to the hospital to give us many in-services on what her model involved and how to get it operational on our units. She herself was interesting, and many of her ideas were interesting and relevant, yet there was little enthusiasm for her model among the middle-management group or the unit nurses. This was attributed, at the time, to a natural anxiety about trying anything new, but in reality, the era of "nursing models" was drawing to a close by this time, and enthusiasm for such models was ebbing nationally. The hospital had also earlier adopted a particular nursing theory as the basis for its nursing practice, and it had been a failure (see Sketch # 28.)

So, to many people, the time and energy it would require to fully implement the system were simply not worth the end result, as all of these models were quite competitive with each other and each required rigid fidelity.

Most nurses looked at these models as too much value to be lost and too little value to be gained.

Eventually the effort to introduce this model lost steam and was abandoned.

On the other hand, in 1985 the nursing department decided that all of the hospital's unit managers should become credentialed as Psychiatric Clinical Nurse Specialists, and that was a very successful project. Clinical Nurse Specialist (CNS) was the new credentialing thrust in nursing at the time, and although the credential itself as a clinical role faded away after a few years, it led eventually to define a successful nurse role with prescriptive rights.

To become a CNS, nurses with graduate nursing degrees were required to take an exam. All managers at the hospital already had graduate degrees, so we were all eligible to take the exam, and we were all enthusiastic about it. The exam itself was difficult, and I only scraped through, but we were all pleased when we got our CNS certificates, feeling that we were not only advancing our own careers, but also playing a part in advancing professional nursing.

Being a CNS later enabled me to be credentialed into the medical staff at an Ohio hospital. I believed this to be important in having nursing recognized as a true health profession, as well as giving nursing input into important clinical/administrative discussions and decisions.

Thoughts: Regarding the Marker Model project: it is healthy and necessary for nursing departments to be periodically engaged in projects that are seen by everyone as enhancing the quality of nursing care. It helps nurses' morale to be actively involved in improving patient care, while there is nothing deadlier for nurses' morale than for them to see themselves in a stagnant culture where nothing new will ever happen.

In this case, most nurses saw the project as not being one that would actually improve patient care on the unit; it was really being done for nonclinical reasons. It was then doomed to failure no matter how much time and energy was devoted to it.

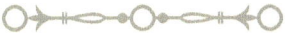

Regarding the CNS project: when we became CNSs, new career options inevitably opened up for us beyond our current hospital. These opportunities might have not been there otherwise. At face value, it would seem strange for a hospital to be almost encouraging good employees to leave, but the opposite was actually true. For when a nursing department develops a culture that encourages nurses to go as far in their careers as they want to go, then that is a culture that people enjoy being a part of.

People will inevitably leave no matter what, but their places will always be quickly filled by good people attracted by an environment in which they are encouraged to explore and fulfill their own professional potential and ambitions.

Nursing departments in academic settings can create this culture almost naturally, while it is difficult for nursing departments in nonacademic settings to replicate it.

Sketch # 54

While it is important to avoid a sense of stagnation on a unit, I think that it's also important to create a sense of tradition, as this can help reinforce to staff members that what they are doing is good, is proven, and is worth continuing to do.

Sometimes this can be done concretely. It can be as simple as someone bringing in some food at staff meetings on a rotating basis, and sometimes it can be done more symbolically.

The poet Robert Lowell had been a patient on this unit several times in the past, and in 1959 had written "Waking in the Blue," (13) a poem about everyday life on the unit. At Christmas staff parties we read this poem. It seemed to me to be a wonderful confirmation to staff members that the work that they were doing had genuine meaning—so much so that it was even worth writing fine poetry about!

Thought: Managers should look for every way to help staff members feel proud about their everyday work.

Sketch # 55

We had a weekly staff meeting at change-of-shift time on Wednesdays, the sort of meeting very familiar to every nurse in every psychiatric hospital. A consistent theme at these meetings was a complaint that I filled the empty beds on the unit too quickly, so that the unit was pretty much always at full capacity.

As I outlined in Sketch # 45, my experience had been that, when a unit makes as its unspoken policy to always try to keep some empty beds and to avoid some admissions if possible, this eventually has a corrosive effect on the general sense of professionalism on the unit. Also, admissions are what keeps hospitals in business so they can pay the salaries of mental health workers, so it's therefore the role of a unit manager to take admissions whenever clinically possible. Thus, my approach as unit manager was to keep our beds full and also to keep all of our staff positions full. Because of this, the unit was usually pretty busy, but we also had enough regular staff members to be able to safely handle the work.

But, while staff members would say that they could see my position on this, they couldn't help but compare our unit to some other units which might have had a lower percentage of full beds. Empty beds meant quieter shifts, they reasoned, so why didn't we do as the other units did? The temptation to cast our eyes elsewhere to make sure that someone else isn't getting a better deal than we are is simply irresistible to all of us.

And so, at the weekly staff meeting I would frequently be asked in different ways why I was being mean and making them work harder than staff members on other units. It was an issue that apparently could never be resolved.

In 1992, I left the hospital to work in a California hospital. We had a last staff meeting in which many people said how much they had enjoyed working with me on the unit. Some even told me that it was the best experience they had ever had. After a while I said, "I'm very thankful for the kind things you've said, and I've also had a great time working with all of you. But for the past few years, at this same meeting, you've many times voiced unhappiness about some of the ways in which I've run the unit. And now you're saying it was all good. I can't figure that out. Why have the complaints now turned to compliments?"

There was a long silence. Then a staff nurse quietly said, "We always actually liked it, but we just didn't want you to stop trying."

Thought: Line staff workers have little ability to control the circumstances of their work lives. They depend to a large extent on their direct manager to reasonably protect them and to create an environment in which they can do their work as well as it can be done. So, line staff workers feel that they have to keep pressure on their manager to do this even when things are going well, out of fear that the manager will become complacent and lose interest in them.

For managers who might be wondering why their staff members complain even when things appear to be going well, there may be cause to worry or there may not be. For, in complaining, staff may be just "doing their job." They may well appreciate what their manager is doing, but they still see themselves as needing to keep the boss on his or her toes.

I later saw this dynamic paralleled in regular meetings of middle nurse managers when I was in an executive nursing role.

CHAPTER 9

A California Hospital

Sketch # 56

In 1992, the Department of Psychiatry at the California hospital that I moved to was in the middle of the same philosophical shift that many psychiatric services were. The existing inpatient unit was, and had been for many years, an open-door, psychosocial, milieu-therapy oriented one, led by Dr. Y. I., a national leader of the existential psychotherapy movement. The nursing staff members were very committed and enthusiastic about this model and their unit.

But the times were changing. The unit was running an unacceptably low patient census, so with Dr. I. retiring at this time, the model was being replaced by the biological psychiatry model endorsed by Dr. S. A.

As part of this transition, the existing unit was going to be closed, and a new locked unit opened within the main general hospital complex. My role was defined as clinical psychiatric specialist, with the initial emphasis on formulating new policies and procedures appropriate to the care of acutely ill mood-disordered patients, and of educating the nursing staff on these new policies and procedures.

The staff members were mainly experienced RNs and were clearly ambivalent about the change of direction their program was taking. They had enjoyed their work for many years and were very fond of their old unit. At the same time, they were aware of the changes taking place in psychiatry and knew that changes would have to be made. Remaining at the hospital was important to them all, and, encouraged by their manager, they accepted the change and became actively involved in learning what they needed to know when the new unit opened.

The unit itself was unlike anything ever seen in the hospital. It was locked, but there was stair access to an attractive outside courtyard and fountain, for both fresh air and smoking breaks (still an important part of patient life at that time). For patient safety, this staircase had to be enclosed with unattractive fencing.

So the psychiatric nursing staff eventually came to terms with the changes, even though there certainly was some trepidation about working with acute, involuntary, patients where physical safety would be much more of an issue in their working lives than it had been up to this point. And this trepidation was shared by many in the general hospital.

Thought: Even though this marked change in clinical direction at the hospital was inevitable, it was equally inevitable that it would evoke anxiety, if not outright fear, in the unit staff members and in others throughout the hospital. In theory, education would probably be viewed as being the main factor in allaying these fears, but in reality, experience in doing it alone would be what worked.

The role of the nurse manager P. C. was absolutely crucial in encouraging the unit nurses to accept and buy into the new unit. In their hearts, these staff members dearly wished that their old unit didn't have to close, and they looked carefully at their manager to see what her position was going to be, as they knew that she felt as they did. Her saying, in effect, "Let's just do it!" made all of the difference in making a successful transition.

Before Dr. I. retired, I was excited to have the opportunity of observing him leading a patient group on the unit.

The whole experience was absolutely fascinating to me. Near the end of the session, Dr. I. gave this feedback to a patient: "I'm trying to feel how you must be feeling about how I'm feeling."

This comment made a particular impression on me, and I couldn't help but think that, when I started psychiatric nursing in the early 1970s, this existential psychotherapy approach would have been very appealing and meaningful to me, while now my main thought was more along the lines of, *I wonder what medications would best help this patient.*

Eras change, and there's simply nothing we can do about that, but we may personally change also, and it's important that we are clearly aware of any changes in our own professional beliefs.

Sketch # 57

This hospital was a great place to be for technology buffs. In 1993 we were introduced to the wonders and horrors of email for the first time, and there were little robots roving round the corridors delivering mail to the units. Sometimes they fell down the stairwells, and children would delight in jumping in front of them causing them to stop, but it was all an advance notice of the coming technological revolution in health care.

Thought: Technology has never been one of my strong points, but I could certainly see the strength of emails in helping to eliminate any confusion regarding what people were asking other people to do.

When conversations were spoken, people could later claim that the other person didn't say what he or she claimed to have said, but a written email eliminated that possibility just as the old "hard copy" memo did, only electronic mail was a lot easier. On the other hand, some people used email as a means of getting others to commit themselves in writing to something that they later wished they hadn't.

Either way, the value of emails in "leaving a paper trail" quickly became obvious to people, and it equally quickly became obvious that no one should ever write an email when angry. That's a sure way of saying something that will later be regretted. My advice is to wait until the next day to write an email when anger clouds the situation, or at least wait for a few hours to cool off a bit.

When email first came out, some administrators made the mistake of thinking that all they had to do from that point on was to sit at their desks and send emails to people. They thought that they didn't need to actually talk with anyone person to person any more. This was a serious error, of course, as many people end up basically ignoring what they are told in an email unless they also believe that that the sender is also genuinely involved with them and cares about them, and only interpersonal contact can do that.

I tended to write long emails, as new ideas would come into my head as I wrote, but the truth is that most people reading the mails probably stopped reading after the first two paragraphs or so. I learned that a two-minute person-to-person conversation was probably more productive for me than a carefully crafted email that took me fifteen minutes to write.

Seeing these sorts of technological advances that I simply hadn't imagined as ever being possible made me very aware that, for the rest of my career, I would have to make a special effort to try to keep up with the inevitable further changes. I had a brain that could be filled with wonder at these advances but one that couldn't necessarily master them. But, as I learned later, a good secretary can paper over many technological cracks.

Sketch # 58

A few months after the unit opened, a man in his early thirties was admitted for evaluation and treatment of an apparent mood disorder.

Early one morning, I was walking down the unit to my office, and this man was one of several patients gathered around the nursing station. If possible, I always said hello to patients as I walked along and hoped to be able to do so for this patient, as he was our most recent admission and I wanted to help make him feel comfortable on the unit.

But he was talking, apparently quite cheerfully, to another staff member, so I walked on. Staff members reported that he appeared relaxed and in no distress during breakfast and afterwards.

About two hours later I was again walking down to my office when I heard a small voice at the other end of the unit say, "Help!" It wasn't loud, and there were lots of other noises on the unit, but it was a frightened, frightening voice that cut through everything and stopped me in my tracks. A second later came another small, bone-chilling "Help!"

There are times that mental health workers know they may safely go rather leisurely toward an incident because they know pretty much what is going on and they don't want to contribute any more drama to an already-overblown situation. And there are times when they know they must just run as fast as they can. The tone of the nurse's voice alone made this an incident that prodded me to run just as fast as I could.

The nurse who had called had been doing patient safety checks on the unit and had discovered the patient slumped on the floor with a torn pillowcase wound tightly around his neck and then attached to the door handle (an unusual but quite possible suicide method.)

We cut the pillow case and successfully performed CPR.

Thoughts: We usually think of mood disordered patients as cycling from manic excitement to suicidal depression over weeks, months, or even years. But uncontrolled rapid cycling such as this patient had is scarily different. The cycling can happen in hours, or even fractions of hours.

Patients sometimes talk in terms of a black cloud quickly and unexpectedly descending over them or of a black hole into which they descend. They are powerless to resist these phenomena or alert anyone that they are experiencing them. Borrowing from Dr. Johnson, Winston Churchill referred to these dreaded periods as his "black dog" visits.

Normally, patients who are assessed as being suicide risks are put on special observation of some sort. But, at any given time, with true rapid cycling, there may not be anything in the patient's presentation to make anyone think that there is a suicide risk. But thirty minutes later it may be a quite different matter

So, whenever nurses hear the term "rapid cycling" applied to a patient, they should prick up their ears, find out from the other treatment team members exactly what that means in that specific case, and make sure that all of the nurses know what it means.

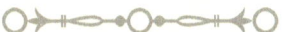

A suicide attempt, successful or not, is the dread in every psychiatric nurse's heart. Most nurses worry about being assaulted by an agitated patient, but having a suicide attempt on their unit, on their shift, is the thing above everything else that they don't want to happen. Many of our policies, procedures, and protocols, and much of our training revolve around preventing that one thing—a suicide attempt.

I have known grizzled, veteran line staff personnel who were first responders to a patient who cut her wrists in a bath. They still teared up when they talked about it ten years afterwards. There's nothing worse for psychiatric nursing staff.

And yet sometimes suicides and suicide attempts happen. They are rare, thank goodness, but they do happen, as patients who have decided to die can sometimes find ways of killing themselves that we simply have not thought of as being possible at that time. All nurses can do is to review them as thoroughly as they can and learn from them.

But nurses should never believe that their unit is perfectly safe with regard to suicide risks, because it's not (see Sketch # 23). Nurses who think about or see anything that is worrisome must make sure to put their concerns in writing (email is fine) to their supervisors and treatment team members.

When there is a suicide or suicide attempt on a unit, staff members very often second-guess themselves in terms of things that they did or didn't do that might have obviated the attempt. In my case, I couldn't help wondering. If I had waited until the patient had finished his talk with the nurse, and then said hello to him and asked him how he was, could this somehow have created some sort of human bond that could have helped him to fight off his black cloud?

This is magical thinking, of course, but it's inevitable that everyone working with a patient who makes a suicide attempt will ponder on his or her own: "If only I'd…" And this will continue for a long time afterwards. Talking about it with each other is the only way to understand that everyone is probably feeling the same way, and that no one is the awful nurse who should quit psychiatry immediately.

Sketch # 59

I was becoming more and more interested in nursing management, and how far I might go as a manager, so I audited a local university evening class, "Aspects of Leadership," in which a widely diverse group of people (from a big-city police chief to a college basketball coach) in leadership positions in their chosen fields talked about what qualities they found to be most important to them in performing their duties. I was starting to think that my future career probably lay in administration, and that raised the question of leadership, about which I still had considerable ambivalence. But before I committed myself to a career in administration, I wanted to do whatever I could to get some clues regarding whether I might end up being a good leader or a bad one.

Later on, when I had been offered my first executive nurse position at a hospital in Massachusetts, I similarly audited an evening class at a Cambridge university on "Ethics and the Law." In this case, I had heard from a number of nursing friends that, at the hospital I was going to, I might "see things that I hadn't seen before," so I was trying to be at least theoretically prepared for the worst before I went. It was a great course, but as it turned out, what I saw there was pretty much what I had seen at a number of other hospitals.

Thought: Nurses who are trying to figure out what they are going to do for their next job or the rest of their career should take advantage of whatever is available to them to help guide them. In these cases, I was able to attend some interesting classes at some pretty good schools, and I somewhat shamefacedly included them in my resume!

CHAPTER 10

A North Shore, Massachusetts, Hospital

Sketch # 60

I returned to Boston and started work in 1994 as a unit manager for one of the psychiatric units at a general hospital in the northern suburbs of Boston with a distant view of the Boston skyline. The local town had the highest average population age in the country at that time, so the general side of the hospital was dealing with an unusually large number of patients who had Medicare/Medicaid as their primary funding. The result was that the hospital was in some financial jeopardy.

The psychiatric services consisted of two inpatient units and a small partial hospital clinic, and it was the sole money-making program in the hospital. (In a partial hospital program, patients attend therapy programs during the day and go home at night.)

It was run by a for-profit company hired by the hospital, an arrangement that I found to be perfectly workable for patients and staff alike. I had some initial concerns that the company might want to cut corners with patient care and staffing levels in order to make more money, but they put no more pressure on me as a unit manager to do that than had any of the not-for-profit or public hospitals that I had worked for.

My only real complaint was that we could never get good enough ventilation equipment installed in the room used for patient smoking breaks. We did get some new equipment, but no matter what, we could never get rid of those nicotine stains dripping down the walls! At that time, I still considered it essential to allow psychiatric patients to have regular smoking breaks, believing that not doing so would inevitably result in agitation and violent behaviors. So my emphasis then was on trying to clean up the filthy smoking room rather than abolish it. It was another ten years before I figured out that my belief about patients clinically needing to smoke was actually wrong.

As the financial situation for the hospital gradually worsened, it was announced that some consultants from Texas were coming to review the psychiatric program, with the result that a month later I found myself manager of both units and the partial hospitalization program.

Thought: Whenever psychiatric staff members are told that "some consultants from Texas" are coming to review their program, it may be time to start checking the classified ads! They're always from Texas, it seems!

And nurses should keep in mind the possibility that what they currently regard as being inviolable truths in their work may later turn out to be false.

Sketch # 61

At this hospital, the on-site weekend and holiday supervisory coverage was provided by a mix of the unit managers and the central staffing office supervisors.

As the psychiatric services were not actually administered by the hospital itself, the psychiatric unit managers had traditionally not been included in this rotation. However, at some point, the managers of the medical-surgical units, the ER, and other groups started to complain that, since they had to cover the psychiatric units on their weekends, then we should provide similar coverage to their units.

This was difficult to argue against, though I knew that I could offer little in the way of meaningful clinical advice or direction to nurses on the general units. The other managers pointed out that they felt the same way when they worked on the psychiatric units.

But it all went well, largely because the staff nurses on the medical-surgical units could probably see a "deer-in-the-headlights" look on my face when I walked on their unit, and they were kind enough not to ask me anything that they figured was probably beyond my ken. The charge nurses would usually tell me that everything was just fine on their units or give me a very abbreviated report. I would nod sagely, we would both smile, and I would go on to the next unit.

Thought: Nurses who find themselves in administrative situations that put them out of their depth clinically must resist the temptation to act as if they have everything under control. There's no shame in not knowing the nursing care of every specialty in detail. Unit nurses don't need administrators to clinically know what they already know; they only need administrators to know what to do administratively if that requirement ever arises.

Sketch # 62

During a regular weekly staff meeting, we were talking about how best to work with a patient who was seriously disrupting the unit, and his psychiatrist made the comment, "Unless I can definitely prove otherwise, I believe everything that my patients tell me."

Even though he explained that this was the way he had been trained to form the basis of his relationship with patients, the rest of us were astonished at this statement, as it seemed perfectly obvious to us that having treatment team members fully believing the often-bizarre delusions that only patients themselves usually believed to be true would be a sure route to chaos on the unit.

Yet the psychiatrist was a good one who worked well with the patients and was well regarded by the unit nursing staff, and we were simply vexed regarding why a competent clinical professional would be making such an apparently outlandish statement.

Nothing was resolved further at the meeting, but it stuck with me for a long time that there must be some sense to his apparently nonsensical statement even if I couldn't see it at that point, as he was a good psychiatrist.

Eventually I arrived at my own conclusion regarding what he was talking about, though I have no idea whether it was aligned with what he himself meant!

That was when I came to realize the simple truth that, when patients explain their delusions, no matter how bizarre and impossible they are, it will destroy any possibility of an effective nurse-patient relationship if nurses simply dismiss what the patients are telling them, or, even worse, perhaps even argue with them about the delusion.

When patients explain their psychotic thinking, whether what they are saying is, strictly speaking, right or wrong is irrelevant. What is important is that this is where the patients are coming from and this is their only way of giving others any clues as to where that is. And if nurses don't accept where psychotic patients are coming from, then there is no possibility of any understanding developing on the part of the nurses, or trust developing on the part of the patients.

For no matter what crazy ideas patients talk to their nurses about, that is where they are, and that has to be accepted even if the delusion itself is not believed. Nurses can look for clues as to whether the delusions mask anger or depression or other symptoms. And nurses can address that with patients, but nurses must not openly dismiss what is clearly important to patients themselves if they hope to develop some positive working relationship with them.

Thought: What is going on inside a psychotic patient's mind is chaos, so inevitably what they often tell those who care for and treat them is chaotic and makes no apparent sense.

But it's all that the patient is capable of giving anyone at that point, so nurses must accept it as such. Patients certainly shouldn't be encouraged by nurses to talk about their delusions, but if that's all patients have to offer, then that's what nurses should take. Nurses may patiently listen to the same psychotic ideas day after day without any apparent impact on their patients' thinking, but what they are doing is slowly giving their patients some notion that they are genuinely interested in them and that they may be someone in whom they can have some degree of trust and confidence (as with Dr. S. B. in Sketch # 12.)

Even in the era of biological psychiatry, the art of working collaboratively with patients must remain a vital part of the psychiatric nurse's repertoire.

There is a definite negative factor in dismissing or arguing with patients over their delusions, for once a listener starts doing that, paranoid patients' antennae are immediately alerted, and nurses sometimes then end up being incorporated into the delusion.

Sketch # 63

While I was at this hospital, I worked for one semester on the adjunct faculty of the college of nursing of a Boston university. As with a lot of such positions, I heard about it from another nurse whom I had worked with in the past, and who was herself now leaving that faculty position and was helpfully looking for someone as a replacement.

Doing my graduate work had put me off the idea of ever going into education full time, but this was just one evening a week working as a clinical instructor of undergraduate students doing their psychiatric rotation at the Boston VA Hospital.

And I liked it. I liked just talking with each student individually for twenty minutes about his or her assigned patient. Most of these students had no intention of going into psychiatric nursing when they graduated, and like many student nurses, they had an actual dread of their psychiatric rotation, so they would ask questions and raise issues that I hadn't thought of before.

Wonderful and Weird

Up to this point, I had primarily worked with nurses who liked psychiatry, and it was interesting to hear other points of view.

My next job took up all of my time and energy, so I stopped the adjunct faculty work at that point. But enjoying this brief time with students put the idea in the back of my mind that this might be something to come back to at some point in the future.

Thought: Almost everyone who works with students finds it interesting and stimulating, so everyone should give it a try whenever the opportunity ever presents itself.

This hospital closed in 1999.

CHAPTER 11

A Massachusetts State Hospital

Sketch # 64

When I was at the North Shore hospital, I noticed that the director of nursing position at a Massachusetts state hospital had opened up, and I found myself intrigued by that. Much of my interest was due to simple ambition on my part: to my surprise, I had found that I enjoyed nursing management, and having made that step, I was curious about how far I could go in that field. Middle managers can make significant differences in the quality of care that their patients receive on their unit, and to the satisfaction of their staff. So, by extrapolation, I figured that the DON should be able to do the same except for a whole hospital rather than just a single unit.

So I applied and got the job, starting in 1995.

This hospital was part of the Massachusetts Department of Mental Health system, the first such hospital in the state when it opened in 1833. Many of the old Gothic Revival Kirkbride-style buildings were still present despite a recent fire, including the administration building and clock tower. These buildings were very striking, but also pretty creepy looking, as if they were really props in a horror movie.

There was also a 1904 building that had been the old nurse training school established by Linda Richards, "the first trained nurse in America." Later in her career, Richards became interested in psychiatric nursing and created training schools in several state hospitals, including this one. She deliberately established these in public asylums as she felt that the need was greatest there, with many of the private psychiatric hospitals affiliated with general hospitals already having their own nurse training schools and thereby being able to provide much higher standards of nursing to their patients (14.) An old grey stone Victorian building, which had served as apartments for nurses working at the hospital, was still in very good condition, though unused.

The actual patient units and administrative offices now being used were in a plain, boxy 1950s building next to the old asylum buildings.

Thought: Some jobs I had taken and felt just fine, but no more. In this case, I just loved the feel of the whole place.

Up to this time, I had never viewed myself as being a "leader"; rather, I had, during all of my adult life, viewed leaders of all sorts with suspicion, and never imagined myself in that role myself. Middle managers are the leaders of the nursing staff on their units, but they can still avoid thinking of themselves as "real" leaders because there's still at least one nurse above them in the organizational chart telling you what to do. But there's no other nurse above those who agree to take a director of nursing position. Directors of nursing must brush away all of their previous ambivalences and accept their responsibilities as leaders. They can look back on the leaders that they have worked for and focus on the facets of their work that they have admired and those that they have been critical of, and only hope that they have learned well. Accepting leadership is just part of growing up, sort of like becoming a parent.

Sketch # 65

During my job interview, I was somewhat surprised to find that one of the people interviewing me was a union official. Years before, I probably would have thought that this was a great idea, but now I was thinking to myself, *Why does the union have a say in who gets placed in executive management positions? Will I have a similar say in elections for union executive positions?*

When I started working there, I was additionally surprised to discover that all of the supervisors and unit managers at the hospital were mandated to be union members. This meant that they could not be involved in disciplining staff who reported to them as they were fellow union members. The only people in the entire nursing department who were not in the union were the three assistant directors of nursing and myself, and the reason there were three ADONs rather than the usual one was that they had to do all of the disciplining. It was an extraordinary situation.

Somewhat unusually, the hospital was not run by a chief executive officer. That role had been downgraded to a chief operating officer position. While this COO had the responsibility of running the hospital, the real power lay with an area director, a political appointee who worked from a suite in the hospital.

Thought: Despite what I regard as their drawbacks regarding professional nursing (see Sketch # 7), my experience has been that unions are necessary in public hospitals to protect staff from the unpredictable but inevitable changes of political winds. And good working relations between management and unions are very important if hospitals are going to operate in the best interests of patients and staff members.

But there must inevitably be some tension between management and unions in order to have a healthy organization, as they have different functions. Management has the responsibility to do what it believes is in the best interests of the whole hospital and possibly beyond, while unions have the responsibility to do what they believe is in the best interests of their members and possibly beyond. These goals are not always the same, which in some cases may lead to conflict, which is then resolved by defined processes.

This inherent tension between management and unions is necessary in order to produce good outcomes. But when the balance is skewed by hospital management being viewed with suspicion by its own governing body while unions are favored for political purposes by having even middle management positions unionized, then the system becomes dysfunctional.

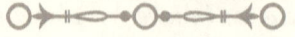

I was surprised but also amused to learn soon after I got to the hospital that one of the assistant director of nurses had two unwritten duties: to check the local paper every day to see if any of the nursing staff had been recently arrested, and also to scan the hospital's parking lots in the late morning to see if there were any "repo" vans cruising around looking for cars of staff members who might be in payment default.

At first this made me glad that I had taken that "ethics and the law" course, but over the next few months, it became apparent that these tasks were more in the nature of carrying on by habit and interest something that had probably once been a useful exercise, and was now probably not absolutely necessary.

Sketch # 66

In the preceding years, the hospital had been the subject of federal and state investigations regarding allegations of patient abuse, and the nurses still working there were almost worn out by the shadows of doubt being constantly cast over their professionalism.

So I thought that my most immediate focus should be on doing something that would make these nurses proud rather than ashamed to say that they worked at the hospital.

We therefore organized a nursing conference entitled: "Meeting the Challenge of Health Care Reform." We held it at the hospital, and it featured Leah Curtin, the nationally recognized commentator on nursing issues and editor of *Nursing Management* magazine. My hope was that seeing and being with hundreds of other nurses who had paid good money to come to a conference at their hospital would give our nurses some confidence that their hospital wasn't the backwater that they feared it was and that it might actually have something to offer in terms of professional nursing.

The conference was an enjoyable one and was well attended. Leah Curtin was funny, insightful, and challenging.

I followed up the conference by having a series of talks on the history of nursing and psychiatry. My hope, again, was to help our nurses raise their professional morale by remembering where psychiatric nursing came from, and by seeing the historically important role that their hospital had played in caring for the mentally ill.

Thought: Looking at a staff nurse's everyday work in a state hospital, with its never-ending problems and frustrations, it is easy to lose sight of the grandeur of the role. I've never worked in a hospital, even the best ones, where nurses happily tell their managers how good their morale is (see Sketch # 47). It just doesn't happen that way, as on any given day their work appears to be the same old struggle. But people in nursing management have a responsibility to do things that they believe will help build and reinforce nurses' professional pride, while never expecting them to tell their managers that their morale is now "good" as a result of what their managers have done.

Those in executive management (and their bosses!) must end up being their own judges as to whether or not they are doing a good job, as so much of the input offered by others has some agenda. The key is to always strive to do the right things for the right reasons.

Sketch # 67

The hospital COO, K. B., had come from the retail sector, a somewhat unusual background. I liked him a lot. He was energetic, smart, and cynical. Plus, he quickly trusted me enough to let me do what I thought was best regarding nursing issues.

He wasn't completely trusted by the hospital staff, as they never quite knew what he was up to.

For instance, he himself once started a rumor that, at random nights, he would go to a nearby hill and watch through a telescope to see if anyone on the third shift was sleeping. He never actually did it, but he reasoned that, if the staff believed that he did, that would be enough to play a part in keeping them awake!

On another occasion, he discovered some serious fraud on the part of a well-established executive manager at the hospital. The two of them had apparently been talking about a college that the other manager had said he had attended when the COO noticed some discrepancies in his description of the campus. Unknown to the manager, he had gone there once himself for a conference. He then checked the manager's entire resume and found that he had actually never attended two of the colleges that he claimed to have attended, so he couldn't have any degrees from them.

Having a COO who didn't hesitate to dig into things if he thought that something might not be right just wasn't what people at the hospital expected, especially if it involved a senior administrator, as most staff members almost automatically assumed that the rules were different for them.

Thoughts: Life is much easier for staff members when they feel their supervisor trusts them. And if staff members trust their supervisors, all the better. Actively liking one another isn't at all necessary in order to have a good working relationship with supervisors or peers, but if it happens, then life is truly good!

Fraud in health care is sadly not that rare. It usually takes the form of people falsely claiming to have academic qualifications that are required for a particular position. Human resource employees simply have to check these claims thoroughly, no matter how appealing and trustworthy a candidate may appear to be during an interview.

But those who obtain positions through fraudulent claims can still do their jobs well, and in this case, the executive did many aspects of his job well.

One thing in particular that I learned from him was how to handle the masses of emails that I always got. Over the course of the day, I would get between seventy and a hundred on the average, and even if I had sorted through them all by the end of my day, there would often be around thirty-five or so more when I got to work at 7:30 in the morning. My usual routine was to go through a few and then start to attend to other things, such as morning report to the COO, a routine which would then result in my spending the rest of the day struggling to get through the rest of the emails, including the new ones, as best I could.

This other executive usually came in at about the same time I did, but after about thirty minutes, he would be wandering about the corridors of the administration building as if he had nothing to do. I asked him what he did with his emails, as it was a constant struggle for me to keep up with them, particularly the mass that awaited me each morning. He replied that he made it his strict policy never to do anything else after he had arrived at work until he had first dealt with all of his emails, as only by doing this could he keep up with the everyday workload that awaited him. I found that this to be generally good advice for myself also, though there were inevitably days when I simply couldn't do it that way.

I also tended to have a pile of unprocessed mail on my desk, and one day I was talking with another executive about how annoying this was to me. He said that the same thing happened to him, and that his way of dealing with it was this: every six months, he simply took the bottom half of the pile and threw it away without looking at it. His logic was that anything that hadn't been dealt with after six months either wasn't important or had been dealt with through some other channel. He emphasized that he never looked at anything; otherwise, he would find a reason not to throw it away. His advice: Just grab a handful and throw it away unseen!

It made perfect sense to me, and I did try it several times without any disasters, but on the whole, my nerve broke about doing it, and my pile usually remained, to be dealt with at a later date.

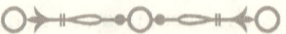

In the administrative building at the hospital, there was an old oil painting in one of the rooms. Nobody knew who it was or gave it any thought. Yet, it was a painting of Clara Barton, quite likely a contemporary one, the noted nurse leader from the American Civil War, and founder of the American Red Cross. She had been born and raised at a nearby town. It was probably worth some good money, but there it was, quite unacknowledged. It made me wonder what else of value and interest might be on display, or more likely in storage, in these old public hospitals— items that, through simple neglect, might well end up being stolen or just thrown away.

Sketch # 68

When I started working at the hospital, I went round all of the units on all of the shifts to introduce myself. Most often, staff members were polite but reserved, giving me a break my first time around, I figured, keeping their real thoughts for the second time.

On the second shift, however, there was one mental health worker who strode confidently up to me, introduced himself, shook my hand firmly, and heartily welcomed me to the hospital. He told me that WSH was a great place to work. He was in his late forties and had been at the hospital for several years.

About a year later, another staff member found him having sex with a young female patient in a side room on the unit. The patient told the police that she had been having sex with him two to three times a week for the past two years. She said that she didn't really want to do it, but that he was very persistent, and while he didn't directly threaten her, she didn't want to say no in case there were any bad consequences for her.

Other staff members said that they'd had some suspicions about what was going on for some time, as he had told them that he was talking to the patient about some of her personal issues, but he only seemed to want to talk to her after the shift supervisor had left the unit on her once-a-shift visit. Yet, they didn't say anything about it to the supervisor at the time, despite their suspicions.

Thoughts: The last thing that I'd want to deter would be a friendly staff member from saying hello to me, but it was interesting that the person who made himself most noticeable when meeting his new DON was the one person who had the most to conceal. "Hiding in plain sight" is an expression worth remembering.

After incidents like this, staff members often share a flood of things that the staff member in question had said or done that had aroused their suspicions. And when they are asked why they never said anything to anyone about it, either anonymously or otherwise, the answer is usually that they just weren't certain and didn't want to start false rumors. This may or may not be true, but the instinct of unionized staff is simply to keep quiet until something happens that makes it easier for them to speak up.

Patient abuse like this has undoubtedly been rampant in some psychiatric hospitals, in times not long gone, but in my time, I have found it to consist more of isolated incidents rather than existing as a systemic problem. But unit staff do have a great measure of control over patients, and bad people will always be tempted to take advantage of that control if they think they can get away with it. Managers should always be vigilant about picking up faintly whispered clues that may relate to patient abuse.

Sketch # 69

I wanted to get some small gift for the nursing staff to mark National Nurses Week, so I asked the COO for $300 from the hospital's general fund to buy some coffee mugs with the hospital's logo on them. Since I asked, he agreed, but also said that, in principle, he thought that it was a bad idea, this being his logic: "Even if you have the best of intentions, a lot of your staff's reaction to being given a sixty-cent coffee mug won't be to say thank you. It'll be to say, 'This is all they think of us?' So you're getting little bang for your buck from doing it. But if you stop doing it one year, those same staff will complain even more bitterly: 'Now they don't even bother to give us a stupid coffee mug!' So you find yourself in a situation in which you're spending money on something that gives you no value back, but you can't stop doing it because, if you do, you'll end up in an even worse place than you were when you started. So, it's best not to start it at all."

Thought: I saw his point, but I couldn't help but think that unit nurses so rarely got any concrete signs of appreciation that there could surely be no harm in giving them a mug, a pen, or a keychain once a year.

So I carried on doing it from that year onwards, using hospital money if I could get it, or drug representative donations if I couldn't, or paying for it myself if I had to. I found that, if the small gift had the hospital's name and logo on it, it was better received by nurses than if it had only a generic "National Nurse's Week" on it. So I always had the hospital name and logo put on the small gifts, as I wanted the nurses to not only be proud of being a nurse in general, but also to be proud of being a nurse at that particular hospital.

Sketch # 70

At the hospital, there was a small forensic unit, the first forensic psychiatric unit that I had been involved with. The patients were mainly there on long-term "not guilty by reason of insanity" (NGRI) status. It was strange to see cameras on a hospital unit, though I could certainly understand why the safety features of a forensic unit would necessarily be different from those in a regular psychiatric unit.

Yet, despite the enhanced security precautions, the staffing on the unit had the worst staff-patient ratio and did not include a registered nurse (RN). Instead, a licensed practical nurse (LPN) was the lead nurse on each shift. I couldn't understand why a unit that needed cameras didn't also need an RN. These were all people who, at one time, had been involved in serious, often violent, behaviors, and it seemed to me that they should be having ongoing, accurate assessments with regard to their mental status and safety risk. This would have involved having RNs assigned to the unit.

I was advised by many people, including the regional staff personnel, that this was not necessary as the unit had been quiet for a long time, and since

RNs don't grow on trees in state hospitals, their assignment is a matter of some importance. I therefore did nothing at the time, but I had it in the back of my mind that the issue should be revisited at some point.

Thought: I later learned that the diagnosis of patients in a forensic psychiatric unit does make a big difference regarding how dangerous the unit might be and what the staffing profile should therefore be. Patients with a criminal history who have active paranoid features to their illness, and/or an antisocial personality disorder are simply going to pose more problems than patients with chronic schizophrenia.

Sketch # 71

In 1997, the COO resigned, and I ended up carrying out that role for a few months. As the medical-surgical nurses at Malden Hospital had done when I was acting as their weekend supervisor (Sketch # 53), similarly the other department heads pretty much took care of their own business during this period, probably partly in order not to overload me and partly because they figured that I would be out of my depth with many of their concrete issues anyway.

I did get a chuckle out of thinking of myself as now being in a descendent of the old "superintendent" role of a Victorian asylum.

It was generally a very interesting experience, but the one thing I liked best of all during my time as acting COO involved the Massachusetts Department of Mental Health Games. Periodically, competitive athletic games would be organized, involving patients and staff members from all of the hospitals in the state system. It was sort of an Olympics for state hospitals, with this one being held on the hospital grounds at this hospital. Somewhat to my surprise, some of the long-term patients really got into the spirit of it and spent some time practicing for their events.

Since the games were being held in our hospital grounds, I was the person to give the introductory remarks, and therefore had the opportunity to end those remarks with the exclamation that so many wish they could make just once in their life: *"Let the games begin!"*

Thought: Those who have an opportunity to take on an "acting" role like this should seriously consider it. People will readily forgive anything but the most horrible goof-ups, and there will probably be many new and interesting experiences to be exposed to. It is best to remember that temporary formal power over people who were previously peers will soon be over. Eventually the role will be over, and those who were temporarily elevated will be back with their peers!

This hospital closed in 2009.

CHAPTER 12

A New Hampshire Hospital

Sketch # 72

Without a supportive COO, I found that I was not enjoying my work in the way that I had before, and with little prospect of that changing significantly, in 1997 I took a position as director of patient care services at a hospital in southern New Hampshire.

It was primarily an adult substance abuse hospital, but also included some psychiatry and residential adolescent programs. The hospital had been founded in 1949 primarily to serve New York Alcoholics Anonymous members who needed treatment. AA cofounder, "Dr. Bob" Smith, was apparently due to be their first medical director, but he died before he could take up the position.

In 1997 it was a private for-profit hospital, owned by an entrepreneur in Maryland. It had a formal capacity of 140 beds, but when I was there the daily census varied from fifteen to fifty patients. The owner said that the hospital became profitable when the census was over twenty-five, but at that time, it was losing money and was the subject of reviews from various state agencies involving financial and quality-of-care issues.

On the positive side, it was on the top of a hill in an absolutely beautiful rural mountainous area of New Hampshire, a great place for patients to think about their lives and hopefully recover from their substance abuse.

My role covered all of the clinical departments: nursing, counselling, and social work. My role did not cover the two physicians. Some people advised me not to take the job due to the hospital's troubles, but my experience with for-profit health care at the North Shore hospital had been generally positive, and I took the position with eyes wide open.

The main focus of the hospital when I got there was that a survey was due in a few weeks by the Joint Commission, the national accreditation body for hospitals. There was a general panic about the survey, as there is in every hospital. But in this case, the panic was well justified, for in the day-to-day chaos of the hospital, no one had systematically collected any clinical data for a long time. No minutes had been kept of meetings if meetings had ever been held, and no one was actually even truly familiar with the Joint Commission standards. Everyone knew that failing the survey could be disastrous for the hospital in terms of the cost of fixing any identified problems and of difficulties with insurance companies refusing to pay for admissions to an unaccredited hospital.

But it turned out to be easy! The owner sent in a single RN who was good at quality assurance, and she quickly dug up some data from somewhere and passed out surveys for patients and staff to fill out.

The result was that, within two weeks of her arrival, there was an impressively large colored graph on a tripod by the hospital's main entrance, and an equally impressive array of pie charts, glowing patient testimonials, and mission statements on all of the bulletin boards.

Only one Joint Commission surveyor came, as we were a very small hospital. He must have been very impressed by what he saw, as he not only passed us, he passed us "with commendation," the most prestigious level of accreditation.

We were all pleased to have the survey behind us, but we also knew that our passing at all—never mind "with commendation"—was simply bizarre.

Thought: A survey by the Joint Commission is an event that creates administrative panic even in the best-run hospitals, a panic that steadily rises in intensity as the survey approaches. And, as a DON, a certain panic would grip my soul also. But I always remembered that experience in which the most chaotic hospital that I ever worked at got the best possible survey outcome. It gave me some inner confidence that, if they could pass, then we would pass too.

Sketch # 73

Probably most of the patients were admitted to the hospital by a charmingly old-fashioned method. Usually family members of alcoholics on benders, or alcoholics themselves, would call the hospital and ask for Joe to come. Joe was an old ex-alcoholic who lived nearby. The hospital would tell him where to go to pick up the patient, though he would usually know that anyway, as these were most likely folks who had many prior admissions and whom he knew well. He would then drive off in his old Buick, sometimes hundreds of miles, always coming back safely with the patient, who might be sobering up, or might sometimes have a bottle still in hand.

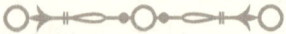

The best explanation by a nurse for not coming to work that I ever heard came while I was at this hospital. One morning the nurse scheduled to be the charge nurse for the day shift called in a panic to say that she was very sorry, but that she would have to call off. This was a rural area, and she kept horses in a barn next to her house. She said that a large pack of coyotes was prowling around the barn and the house, howling away, and that she was afraid that the horses were getting spooked and might break out of the barn if she couldn't calm them down. However, she was also scared to leave her house to tend to the horses, as she was afraid that the coyotes would then attack her, so she was stuck.

It was one of those stories so improbable that it had to be true! (Everything turned out okay, she later reported.)

Thought: Working at this hospital was a chaotic and draining, yet an always-interesting experience, with never a dull day. But when the third

CEO in less than a year announced that all employees would be required to live locally (I lived seventy miles away in Boston), it was time to move on.

I also turned fifty years old while I was at this hospital, and that event made me aware that, up to that time, I had accumulated very little in the way of the savings and pensions that I would need when I retired. For much of my career, I had spent one or two years at several hospitals, with my time at each one ending when I started to think: *That was interesting. Now, what's next?*

So, other than a pension from one hospital I had worked at, I had nothing, and retirement now seemed something that I needed to pay urgent attention to, whereas I hadn't really thought about it at all up to that point.

This hospital closed in 2001.

CHAPTER 13

An Ohio Hospital

Sketch # 74

At a Boston hospital, I had worked with a psychiatrist, Dr. W. D., on several units, and we had enjoyed working together. At this time, he was chief clinical officer (medical director) at a hospital in Ohio, and when he called to ask if I would be interested in interviewing for the director of nursing position there, it was the right thing at the right time.

The hospital was a part of the Ohio Department of Mental Health (ODMH) and traced its history ultimately back to 1821.

That old hospital had been torn down and replaced by a mainly one-story building named after a distinguished volunteer who had unexpectedly dropped dead in the superintendent's office. It was a ramshackle hospital, apparently built in the expectation that new psychiatric medications would eradicate mental illness and therefore render the traditional state hospital unnecessary. Instead, the future of state hospitals was then projected to lie in caring for psycho-geriatric patients.

As it turned out, while those medications certainly helped greatly, they didn't actually cure mental illness. So, instead of the anticipated psycho-geriatric population, the hospital ended up finding itself with about a 75 percent forensic psychiatric population, with most of those having dual mental illness and substance abuse diagnoses.

This meant that a hospital designed to accommodate old folks was now holding primarily people with criminal histories.

Thought: As it is with many other careers, the direction of a career in psychiatric nursing at any given time may be determined by those we happen to know almost more than any other factor. So we must all value our colleagues and burn as few bridges as possible!

And central planners must be careful not to base too many long-term plans on what may turn out to be initially overly optimistic projections.

Sketch # 75

While working with a general psychiatric patient population always brings with it the potential for boundary violations damaging to both patients and staff members, those risks are multiplied when working with a forensic psychiatric population.

With a general psychiatric patient population, the intensity of the professional nurse-patient relationship may result in emotions developing on either side that distort the professional relationship into becoming a personal relationship.

While this remains true for working with forensic psychiatric patients, there is the additional danger that some of these patients (usually those with an additional personality disorder diagnosis) will deliberately attempt to seduce nurses into boundary violations. This is done with the goal of compelling nurses to provide patients with sex or contraband items such as cigarettes, alcohol, and drugs, or actively collaborating in an escape attempt.

The commonest scenario is one in which a young, inexperienced female nurse becomes infatuated with a charming sociopathic patient who pays assiduous attention to her. The sense of excitement and danger that such patients can project to unwary nurses may then sweep all professionalism aside, with the nurses then becoming willing accomplices in the patients' various plans.

But while this is the commonest scenario, there is really no limit to what can happen with this patient population. I knew a middle-aged nurse who became romantically obsessed with a patient much older than herself. He was diagnosed only with paranoid schizophrenia with no personality disorder, and presented with repetitive violent, regressed behavior.

He had killed a man thirty-five years earlier and was now hospitalized on a "not guilty by reason of insanity" (NGRI) status. Despite his dangerous behavior related to his severe chronic mental illness, something in this patient struck such a chord with this nurse that she was willing to jeopardize her professional career in the hope of developing a personal relationship with him.

Who holds the power is always a major factor for nurses working with forensic psychiatric patients. Nurses, of course, have almost all of the legal power, so the strategy of some patients is to steadily erode that power so that they end up controlling the nurses' behavior.

There are rare occasions, however, when predatory nurses take advantage of the power that their position gives them in order to abuse patients. I knew a nurse who forced a male patient in the hospital on a "restoration to competency" (RTC) status to have frequent sex with her, under threat that she would report him as having raped her if he did not comply with her requirements. The patient knew that the nurse would almost certainly be believed in such an accusation, and that he would then be spending a long time in prison, so he agreed to her demands.

Thoughts: Boundary violations and abuses such as these most often occur on the second or third shifts, as professional supervision on those shifts commonly consists of a shift supervisor spending a few minutes on each unit each day. There are usually more staff members present on the first shift, including members of other disciplines and unit managers, so abuses tend to be more quickly recognized on that shift. However, if a nurse is vulnerable to boundary violations, problems can certainly occur on that shift also.

As noted in Sketch #10, all psychiatric and forensic psychiatric hospitals should stress the dangers of nurse-patient boundary violations in both their initial nurse orientation and their continuing nurse education. And they should stress the need for all nurses to be vigilant in noting if such violations start to become evident in either themselves or in a colleague. Again, a vital resource in any education on staff-patient boundaries must involve reading the excellent book *Games that Criminals Play*, by Bud Allen (10)

Whenever a serious violation is revealed, nurses' colleagues regularly say that they had their suspicions for a while, yet they failed to report the situation to their managers or supervisors. Part of the reason for this is simply that they don't want to get a colleague into disciplinary trouble, or fired, and part of it is the forlorn hope that the problem will somehow resolve itself and just go away.

When a staff-patient boundary violation occurs, and other staff members start to become aware of it, they will talk about it amongst themselves yet not raise the issue openly when managers and supervisors are present. But faint clues will still be offered by staff members that something is going wrong, and managers and supervisor should be vigilant in listening for such clues and following up on them.

A boundary violation that can be identified can lead to healthy professional growth on the part of nurses, but this first requires that the nurses involved acknowledge that there is a problem in the first place. And this is often the stumbling block, with nurses often simply denying everything and thus ending up having to be fired.

When I worked as a nursing administrator, I always reported nurses who left my hospital following a serious boundary violation to the appropriate state Board of Nursing. Yet, somewhat worryingly, after a few months it wasn't uncommon to hear that these nurses had simply taken another job at another hospital.

Sketch # 76

Mr. T. died at the hospital when he was ninety-four years old. He had been a patient at the hospital ever since his parents had brought him there as a teenager in the early 1920s, saying that there was something wrong with him and that they couldn't handle his behavior any more. So the doors closed behind him, and that was it for the rest of his life.

He had an official psychiatric diagnosis when he died, but no one really knew what illness he had when he was originally admitted, or if he even had a diagnosis at all. All that was certain was that, by the time medications that might have enabled him to be discharged became available in the 1950s and '60s, he was too rigidly institutionalized to ever be discharged anyway.

By that time, it was a matter of simple human kindness to keep him at the hospital, rather than forcibly trying to discharge him "out of principle," so he stayed there.

He was the last of that generation at the hospital, though old-time nurses did remember others like him.

Thought: Some people might view Mr. T's case as a damning indictment of the old psychiatric hospital system, but I don't. At that time, and before it, families had no way of handling a family member who showed the behaviors of someone with a serious mental illness, so in the end, they took them to the hospital.

But the hospital itself had really no way of effectively treating the patients at all, never mind curing them. All they could do was keep them locked up, try to stop them killing themselves or someone else, and hope for the best. This wasn't a fault of "the system"; the science that could have helped people to do more just didn't exist at the time.

Sketch # 77

Ever since I had started working in psychiatric hospitals, I had taken it for granted that it was a necessary part of life in a psychiatric hospital to allow patients to smoke cigarettes. Overwhelmingly, patients with a major mental illness smoked and appeared to crave smoking above almost anything else, leading mental health workers to believe that not being able to smoke for whatever reason could quickly cause patients to become agitated.

Staff members believed that allowing patients to smoke was vital in maintaining some general sense of stability on their units, and that dispensing tobacco or threatening to withhold it was an important tool in ensuring safe patient behavior.

In short, we all believed that, if tobacco wasn't available to our patients, then the units would quickly descend into violence and chaos.

Some hospitals had open-air smoking porches attached to the units, some had smoking rooms on the units themselves, while others took patients to an open space outside of the main hospital monitored by staff and campus police. A standard patient allowance was something like two cigarettes three times daily, while some hospitals allowed more, some less.

Tobacco itself was the real currency for patients rather than money. It could be traded for food, for sexual favors, for clothes, and so forth, or as the price for not being assaulted. People visiting patients or patients returning from passes would sometimes try to smuggle in contraband tobacco rather than money. The patients' demand for tobacco would also sometimes permeate hospital employees. I have known unit housekeepers to supplement their incomes by selling tobacco to patients, and it would be naïve to think that some nurses didn't also engage in this.

But it was still one of the accepted, indisputable truisms of psychiatric nursing that allowing patients to smoke was absolutely necessary for units to function safely and effectively. No questions asked.

My acceptance of this began to erode in 2004 when I read an article by a psychiatrist describing how his unit had gone smoke-free, emphasizing that none of the disasters predicted by everyone had actually happened. Shortly afterwards, I was at a conference and talked to a director of nursing at another hospital which had just gone smoke-free, and she confirmed that there was none of the violent chaos on their units, as feared by almost everyone of all disciplines.

If patient behavior did not actually seriously deteriorate if a hospital went smoke-free, then there seemed to be little reason not to do it. Without that factor, all that was left was a serious health issue and cause of underground institutional corruption. (Interestingly, however, the incidence of lung cancer in people with schizophrenia who smoke appears to be lower than for people who smoke but do not have schizophrenia.)

So, I asked the CEO if we could go smoke-free, and she agreed.

We gave ourselves nine months to prepare for it, enough time to overcome the inevitable patient and staff resistance through careful explanation and education.

When they were first told about it, patients were angry, but probably not to the degree that I had anticipated. Perhaps they reckoned on getting enough tobacco through the usual contraband routes, or maybe they could only live in the moment and not look too far ahead.

Staff members of all disciplines were initially convinced that going smoke-free would be a disaster with regard to maintaining safe patient behaviors on the units. But some interesting side issues came up that weakened some of this resistance, for if the hospital went smoke-free, then all employees would be included, not only patients. Staff members who smoked would routinely take smoking breaks off the unit during their shifts, and while, in theory, this was subject to contract agreements regarding staff breaks, nonsmoking staff would complain that staff who smoked actually took much more time off the unit than they did. Nonsmoking staff members then saw the hospital going smoke-free as a way of eliminating this abuse and started to support it.

After the nine months, we finally went smoke-free, and while our hearts were certainly in our mouths on that first morning, everything went well. There was no patient violence. Contraband incidents did increase initially, but over the next few months levelled off to the same numbers that we had previously.

Thoughts: Smoking in psychiatric hospitals was one of those issues that we all believed was absolutely necessary and were beyond questioning. But as it turned out, it wasn't necessary at all.

Psychiatric staff should keep open minds for other truisms that may similarly not turn out to be quite as true as always believed. They shouldn't necessarily be deterred by staff resistance if they believe that what they are doing is the right way to go.

Sketch # 78

The medical records department had some old patient admission logs that dated from the 1850s when the hospital opened, to the turn of the twentieth century.

Dementia praecox, the name formerly given to schizophrenia, was listed quite a few times as the admission diagnosis or cause of admission, as one would expect.

But the cause of admission that appeared possibly more often than any other single one was "Disappointment in love."

Victorians were certainly prone to indulging in sentimentality, but even given that, it was intriguing to see it listed so frequently by a diagnosing psychiatrist as a cause of mental illness requiring hospitalization.

These days we would readily say that the breakup of an important relationship, or the failure of a relationship to develop in the first place, could be a major precipitating factor in the development of depression, anxiety, and stress. Similarly, these old logs communicated that disappointment in love had been a major factor in leading to melancholia in patients, only the idea was expressed in a charmingly human way.

Much has been said about the experience of being in love as being a variation of a psychotic state, and certainly the expression of someone being "madly in love" is no accident. Robert Louis Stevenson accurately referred to it as "this pretty madness" (15), for when we are madly in love we see our beloved's face when he or she is not there, and we hear our beloved's voice when he or she is not there. We harbor grandiose ideas about everything related to our beloved that are scarcely any different to a true delusion, while our elated mood, inability to concentrate, and failure to sleep properly similarly mimic a hypomanic state.

Thought: The old diagnosis of melancholia eventually became known as depression, and similarly, the Victorian diagnosis of dementia praecox became known as schizophrenia.

In the 1890s, German psychiatrist Emil Kraepelin assigned the name *dementia praecox* to the illness because he saw it as an organic illness involving a cognitive deterioration in the brain's functioning, commencing in teenagers and young adults.

Swiss psychiatrist Eugen Bleuler believed that Freud's ideas of the psychodynamic causes of neuroses could also be applied to psychoses. He saw the illness not as being the result of organic brain damage, but of the fragmentation and splitting of the patient's thinking processes due to psychological causes, which could then potentially be cured by psychoanalysis. He therefore introduced the term *schizophrenia* in 1908 to emphasize this psychological schism in the mind of the patient.

When I started working at the Boston hospital in the early 1980s, it was still routine for patients diagnosed with schizophrenia to be treated by a psychoanalyst. But in this current era of biological psychiatry, how many clinicians would claim now that schizophrenia is caused by psychological issues?

Would it therefore be legitimate to change the word *schizophrenia* to another one that more accurately portrays our current beliefs about the illness, just as Bleuler changed it in his day?

Or perhaps the term has become so familiar and accepted by us all that what it actually meant to convey to us has become irrelevant.

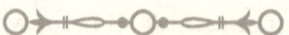

During a quiet evening shift when I was working in my first hospital, the supervisor took me to a basement room where the Victorian-era patient commitment papers were stored. One 1880s document described a patient who was most likely very manic and had assaulted someone on the street for no apparent reason. When asked by the doctor why he had done this, his reply had been: "Because that's how they settle things in America!" This was an early example of the commonly held belief in England that society in the United States was inherently more violent than society in England, and that psychiatric patients in the United States would therefore inevitably be more violent than patients in England. This was a belief that I confirmed after having worked in both countries.

Sketch # 79

When I first worked in the United States as a staff nurse, I was only vaguely aware of the existence of the Joint Commission on Accreditation of Health care Organizations (JCAHO.) Even when a survey was actually happening, it impacted a nurse's daily work very little; it was much more of a management issue than a line staff one.

But in the past thirty years, the Joint Commission has become a dominant feature of everyone's life in health care, from the hospital CEO to the psychiatric mental health worker. Every policy that is written, every meeting that is held, every minute that is kept of those meetings, every clinical or personnel trend that is tracked—the reality is that everyone must always have to ask above almost everything else: "How will this look at the next Joint Commission survey?"

A gradual panic starts to grip everyone in the months before a survey, with each department highly anxious not to be the one to cause the hospital to have a poor survey, or for the hospital to have a poorer survey than other hospitals in the same network.

Whether the time and energy and money spent in this process is an overall positive for health care only time will tell, but meanwhile it's a fact of life that there's no escape from.

We were in the first day of a regular, once every three years survey at the hospital, and it was grinding on in its usual way. I had spent all day with the nurse surveyor, and in the late afternoon, we were walking through the hospital's main corridor as she prepared to leave for the day. In this corridor there were some fiddle-leaf fig plants, donated by an administrative person at the hospital.

She stopped at one of these plants and rubbed a leaf. She commented on it being dusty, which it was, and then went on her way.

I had learned by this time that surveyors never made such comments without having a purpose, even if the subject appeared to have nothing to do with nursing. So when she had gone, I spent twenty minutes washing and shining the leaves of all of the plants.

Sure enough, the first thing that the nurse surveyor did the next morning was to go down that corridor and rub a leaf on another of the plants. She made no comment, but the rest of the survey went well for nursing.

Thoughts: When it comes to publicly funded hospitals particularly, Joint Commission surveyors can basically pick any standard in their manual and nail a hospital with it. The funding and available resources are just so tight that a surveyor has only to start scratching the surface a little before the cracks become painfully evident.

Good surveyors understand this, and rather than vigorously pursuing every possible standard, they will instead try to get some general sense of the prevailing culture of the hospital, to see if the patients are in good hands or not.

In the case of the leaf inspector, she was testing to see how I would respond to her comment that the leaf was dusty, as that response might then provide her with some clues regarding whether our culture was one of fixing identified problems, or of ignoring them.

Staff members should listen carefully to those apparently random or irrelevant comments made by surveyors, as they may be the most important things that they say!

Wonderful and Weird

Sketch # 80

Our assistant director of nursing, R. M., died after a long illness, having worked at the hospital since she became a nurse as a young woman. Everyone had liked and respected her, including people from the non-nursing disciplines.

At that time, the hospital did not have an annual award to recognize outstanding clinicians, so I suggested that the hospital establish such an award in her name. The CEO agreed, so we quickly raised over $1,000 and presented the first award a few months later, consisting of a certificate and $100. The award continues to be the hospital's most prestigious clinical award, many years later.

Thought: Clinical excellence must be recognized in any hospital that has raising clinical standards as one of its goals, but perhaps particularly so in state hospitals, where the culture sometimes tends to be one in which clinicians recognize each other at the unit level but expect only to be taken for granted at the administrative level.

So I was pleased to be able to have a formal recognition of excellence established in the hospital, and I was particularly pleased that this award was named after a nurse. For nurses—the one discipline whose members are with the patients 24/7—often have fingers pointed at them by other disciplines when anything goes wrong clinically, and it was important to emphasize that nursing practice be presented as a clinical model worthy of being emulated by everyone.

Sketch # 81

One afternoon, after I had been in the director of nursing position for about seven years, I was walking down a corridor in the administration building to some committee meeting when an odd thought came to me: *I've set all of the tops spinning that need to be spinning in order for the nursing department to be operating well, but do I truly know if they're still spinning properly or even still spinning at all?*

This was a very worrying thought, as when I had taken the job I had dearly wanted to be an effective DON for the hospital, able to organize good care for the patients, enable job satisfaction for the nursing staff, and represent professional nursing well at the executive level.

Also, in the back of my mind was the knowledge that in the Ohio Department of Mental Health, the nurse executive role was not a particularly secure one, and that there was a steady turnover in people in that position. It was an "at will" position, meaning that a DON could be dismissed for no formal reason other than the CEO wanted it done.

The most obvious thing that I could think of for finding myself at this point was that I had become gradually isolated from what actually happening on the units, and more dependent on drawing my information from purely administrative sources.

So I would routinely go the QA Committee meeting, the Safety Committee meeting, the Morbidity and Mortality Committee, the Medical Staff meeting, the Executive Committee meeting, and the dozen other regular committee meetings. I would then come out of those meetings with lots of data about how many seclusions and restraints we'd had over the past month, how many injuries, how my overtime budget was doing, how many vacant positions we had, and so forth.

But while this data was in itself helpful and necessary, I realized that I hadn't, for example, chatted with Nurses W and X on Unit Y and Z, or had a meeting with the third-shift staff for a long time. Such conversations might well be able to put a vitally different slant to the data that I was getting from the various committees.

In other words, I had gradually fallen into the managerial trap of spending too much of my time in the administration building doing administrative things, while withdrawing from the clinical areas and direct-care staff.

I had weekly meetings with the unit managers and periodic ones with the shift supervisors, and while I had personally hired most of them and on the whole trusted their input to be valid, there was always an inevitable human tendency for them to downplay problems in their own areas of responsibility while emphasizing problems in other areas.

On the other hand, direct-care staff have no trouble pointing out problems on their own unit, as those impact their minute-by-minute lives and are their sole interest.

When I looked back on my work at that hospital, I saw that I had started in the job having monthly meetings with the staff on all three shifts, and had regularly been on the units, but over time, I had scheduled these meetings only every three months, and then only every six months, while my time on the units had become more and more irregular.

Thoughts: Managers can easily fall into this trap if they don't stay consciously aware of it. Going to endless administrative committee meetings becomes very easy and comfortable after a while. Quite likely it's the same people on many of the committees, and it's easy to get to know them well pretty quickly. Committee meeting attendees review important data and do some problem solving, but for much of the time this committee work can be comfortable and rote.

On the other hand, managers who go to the units to talk to staff, or have staff meetings, can expect a lot of complaints about a whole range of issues, some of which they can ultimately do something about, but many of which they can't. Managers may come out of many of those meetings feeling uncomfortable and frustrated, no matter how important they know the input to be.

So, on the one hand, managers have administrative meetings that are often predictable and comfortable, compared to clinical meetings that may be unpredictable and uncomfortable. And as the years go by, the tendency to take the easy road can be very tempting, even though they theoretically know that working through the issues that direct-care staff raise with them is the only way to ensure that the professional nursing goals that they believe in are being met on the units.

That's when managers know that they're probably burning out.

Without these direct meetings with clinical staff, managers can never be sure that they really know what's happening on the units. I had weekly meetings with unit managers and supervisors whom I mostly trusted, but I could still never be certain that they were telling me the whole truth and nothing but the truth about what was happening on their units and shifts, as everyone in every system had his or her own agenda in addition to the stated agendas of the department and hospital.

I realized that the only way I could make sure that the important tops were still spinning in their proper way was to go back to having more regular, frequent direct meetings with unit staff, and to make sure that I visited the units on a more regular basis.

My advice to new executive nurses would be to allot a certain percentage of their weekly time to be in direct contact with unit staff and to be on the units, and to stick to this schedule no matter what the temptations and pressures may be to do otherwise. The percentage doesn't have to be high and may need to be readjusted from time to time as more and more system responsibilities come their way, but they should figure out one that makes sense for them and then make sure that they track that they are meeting it. The percentage that I gave myself at this time was 10 percent. That may not sound like a lot, but it enabled me to learn directly from the horse's mouth and let everyone else know that I didn't rely solely upon their input to know what was going on.

Line nursing staff members don't need—and don't want—to see nurse executives all of the time, they just want to see them in person enough to reassure them that the executive is still interested in them and cares about them.

Sketch # 82

In the early 2000s, the Department of Mental Health, as part of a more general national debate, started to raise the question of whether psychiatric patients should be called patients or should be more properly given some other title.

Wonderful and Weird

The title given to people with a mental illness has a particular significance regarding how they are viewed politically. Politicians with responsibility for health care budgets are well aware that people with serious long-term mental illnesses are unlikely to work for anything other than short periods in their lives, while at the same time, they will require expensive psychiatric services for most of their lives. This means that they will pay very little in taxes themselves, while at the same time they will need a considerable amount of tax payer–funded services.

Politicians are therefore always hopefully looking for any signs that serious mental illness is on the verge of being cured, as that would make a big difference to their budgets. In the absence of an actual cure, the best option that psychiatric administrators can offer to anxious politicians are new treatment models which offer at least some hope of improvement. The title *patient* conjures up to politicians long periods being spent in hospital at an expensive daily rate, so new models try to get around this this by coming up with new titles.

The title *client* had already been around for some time by the early 2000s, with advocates claiming that that patients were clients of health services in the same way that a person might be a client of any other service, and that acceptance of this status would inevitably improve the quality of health services provided to them.

The newer title now being proposed was *consumer*, with again advocates of this title claiming that, if health care providers started to view patients as consumers of their services in the same way that every one of us is a consumer of some service or goods, this would change for the better how health services were provided.

ODMH itself had a brief flirtation with the title *human*, but with that came the prospect of our then referring to inpatient units as inhuman units, and the initial enthusiasm for this faded away before it was put to the test.

Advocates of alternative titles for mentally ill people claimed that the title patient is inherently demeaning and inevitably must lead to abuse of the patient by members of the medical team caring for them, due to the power differential suggested by the title.

In addition to the need to give politicians some hope, these various attempts to eliminate the title patient also represents a reaction by some mental health disciplines against the solidification of the medical-biological model of psychiatry in the 1980s and '90s.

For by 2000 the medical-biological model of mental illness was indisputably recognized as a legitimate research and practice-based model. But there were other health disciplines who felt excluded by this model, including psychologists, social workers, occupational therapists, and psychotherapists among others. These disciplines had all felt much more comfortable in the earlier psychodynamic and therapeutic milieu era of psychiatry and were afraid that they were now being slowly becoming marginalized in the new medical-biological era.

Psychiatric care being established as a medical issue involving primarily doctors, nurses, and patients was something that therefore had to be challenged by the nonmedical disciplines, with that challenge centering around the use of the title patient. For once that title is taken away, then the medical-biological model, in theory at least, becomes open to alternative interpretations.

This in turn gave birth to the "recovery" movement in psychiatry, which stresses the role of the nonmedical disciplines, while not appearing to directly challenge the clinical dominance of the medical-biological model. (Though I did attend an ODMH conference that started with the keynote speaker declaring: "The medical model has failed our consumers ... it is time for a new model, the recovery model...")

"Recovery" was also a positive, encouraging word for politicians to hear, as it suggested the possibility that, with a new treatment model, psychiatric patients might require less funding and might even end up becoming tax payers themselves.

Thoughts: The title client has become a popular one in outpatient psychiatry, but in hospital settings, patients are still properly called patients. Only political administrators still appear refer to patients as consumers.

As our understanding of the chemistry of human thought processes advances, that knowledge will give birth to better and better medications and treatments, but meanwhile, politicians who worry that the cost of psychiatric care is a bottomless pit eating away at their budgets will be periodically offered different words as the next best thing to a cure.

I read an article some years ago in which actual patients were asked what they liked to be referred to as: their number-one choice was client; number two was patient; and a distant third was consumer.

Sketch # 83

One day I got a letter at the hospital from a Kentucky law firm asking if I would be interested in potentially acting as an expert witness in a case that they were involved with. The case involved a man who had voluntarily admitted himself into a Kentucky psychiatric hospital, but he never told his employer that he had done this.

He had therefore ended up being fired on the "no-show no-call" basis. He then sued the hospital, claiming that it was their responsibility—not his—to have informed his employer. The suit specifically named the RN who did his admission as the person who should have called them.

The law firm was representing the hospital in this suit, and one of the attorneys was soliciting my opinion on whether or not I would consider it to be a standard of practice for an admission nurse at my hospital to call an employer to inform him or her of a patient's admission, and if I would act as an expert witness for them should the case come to trial after reviewing the admission documentation.

He added that, even if I decided to not remain involved in the case after reviewing the documents, I would still be paid for any time so spent.

I was intrigued simply because I'd never done anything like that before, and the case appeared to be one in which I had the professional credentials and experience to legitimately give an opinion. However, I also can't rule out the fact that endless TV shows involving "expert witnesses" may have also played a part in flattering my narcissism!

So I agreed to review the documents—a mixture of medical and personnel records—and having done so, agreed to serve as an expert witness should the case come to court.

I didn't give this anymore thought during the several months that went by, but then the attorney gave me a concrete date in a few weeks' time when the trial would start.

At that point, I started to get anxious and half wished that I'd never got involved in the case. I knew that it would be the job of any prosecution attorney to make me look foolish on the witness stand, and having never testified before, I figured that my ending up looking just that way was a real possibility. So I repeatedly pored over all of the HIPAA regulations and the hospital's nursing policies and procedures regarding admission to try to make sure that I could respond to any question that I could imagine being asked.

As the days went by, my initial confidence slowly began to be eroded by anxiety, but the attorney, knowing that this was my first such case, several times gently pointed out to me that I really did know about this sort of stuff—this was my area of expertise. That helped a lot.

Nevertheless, it was to my considerable relief when the attorney called me the day before the trial was due to begin to say that the case had been settled out of court. He thanked me for my involvement and told me that the check was in the mail!

Thought: Most cases like this do end up being settled out of court, and it's quite likely that, in this case, the attorneys always intended to settle and just needed to have the names of "expert witnesses" written down to give some "beef" to their side of the suit, but never intended to actually use them in court.

People who are asked to act as expert witnesses and give evidence in court, while it may be interesting and may pay well, must always remember that they are putting themselves in a situation in which their experience, credentials, and testimony will inevitably be vigorously challenged by clever and experienced attorneys on the other side.

Above all, people should become involved only in cases in which they are very confident themselves that they have the professional experience, credentials, and knowledge relevant to the case.

It may be one of those things that people have to do once to see if they can handle it well, but they should consider their decision carefully, as being humiliated in public isn't something to rush into!

Sketch # 84

I started teaching a graduate course on forensic psychiatric nursing at a Cincinnati university in 2004, and I did that for nine years.

To me, working with graduate students was probably even more fun than working with undergraduates. They're usually older, and therefore more certain about themselves and what they want from life and from nursing. They pretty much know that they're going to get their degree, so they can focus on learning and enjoying the work rather than feeling pressured about grades.

Thought: Nurses have sometimes asked me how soon they should take their master's degree after completing their bachelor's studies. My reply has always been, "A minimum of three years."

I base this on trying to balance two competing factors: One, people tend to find it harder to get back into the flow of academic work the longer they're away from it, so that would suggest going back to school as soon as possible. Two, in order to have a graduate degree actually provide new insights into a nursing practice, nurses need to have a certain amount of real nursing experience to draw on. They can go straight from undergraduate to graduate work and end up with a master's degree. That will certainly help them with their careers, but it won't necessarily help they with advancing their actual practice.

Three years seems to be about the right balance to me.

Of course, many graduate students don't have the luxury of having to make that decision, as they can't go back to school until their children have grown up, or until they have enough money in the bank, among other reasons.

Sketch # 85

I was fired as director of nursing after ten years in that position.

I had never been fired before, and for some time I was consumed by what I regarded as the unfairness of it. I started looking at other jobs, but it soon became apparent that for a sixty-year-old ex-DON, my options were very limited compared to what I had previously been used to. I had been introduced to the staff of the California hospital I had worked in as being the candidate chosen "after a national search," but then I had been forty-three years old and in the prime of my career, and my situation was now simply different seventeen years on.

So, in the time-honored tradition of older, dismissed DONs, I saw out the last of my career as a staff nurse on the night shift.

Thoughts: I wondered a lot about how I would be received by unit staff members now that I would be working alongside them as an equal rather than above them as their administrator. As it turned out, their main concern was that I would act as if I automatically knew more about everything than they did and would therefore expect them to automatically follow what I said without discussing anything with them first.

I was no longer "the boss" and had no administrative power over staff members, but they worried that, instead, I might start to behave in a "big-headed" manner and use my education and experience as a form of power over them.

So simply not acting as if I automatically knew all aspects of unit life and the staff nurse role better than they did, when I obviously didn't, went a long way in helping me to integrate with my new colleagues.

On the whole, I found that actively intervening as a staff nurse in unsafe patient behaviors was not a particular problem for me; all that came back pretty quickly, and I wasn't afraid of it. But what I did have problems with was the practical task of drawing up multiple intramuscular medications quickly for emergency situations. I hadn't done that for twenty-five years, and we were now using medication dispensers rather than just going to a cupboard for the medications, so I was painfully aware of how slow I was at this compared to the other nurses. They were probably aware of it too, as RNs coming to the unit for an emergency would quite often kindly offer to do that part for me of the process for me.

The syringes themselves had been reviewed by the departmental Nurse Practice Committee, and as DON, I had looked them over and approved them, but the obvious turned out to be indeed true—checking something out in the peace and quiet of a private office doesn't necessarily give a person a meaningful indication about how practical it might be in the heat of action.

Sketch # 86

One night I was taking my turn observing a patient who was on a suicide watch. I was sitting in a chair just outside the bedroom door, and the patient was sleeping in the bed closest to the door.

There was a thirty-year-old patient in the bed at the other side of the room, and at one point he got up to use the bathroom. When he was returning to bed, I said, "Goodnight, Mr. Y." to him.

About five minutes later the patient got out of bed again, and slowly started to head out of the room. This in itself was nothing unusual as patients were frequently checking on the unit clock for the time or getting a drink from the unit water bubbler.

There was plenty of room for him to get by my chair, so I stayed sitting in the chair.

Once he was next to me, he started punching me about the head. This continued until I was able to push him away with my feet, and other staff members responded.

He later told my unit colleagues why he had assaulted me: "He made fun of my headless mother!" He said I had done this when I had wished him goodnight. He had a paranoid schizophrenic illness, with fantasies of cutting off his mother's head.

Thoughts: It's a standard axiom in psychiatric nursing to never crack a joke with a paranoid patient, as almost certainly the patient will interpret it in a quite different manner from that which you intend.

And while that is certainly true, this case illustrates that deeply paranoid people are also quite capable of incorporating even the most apparently neutral or inoffensive comments into their delusional systems.

I was angry with myself more than anything for putting myself in a position in which I could be assaulted. I had tried to guess what the patient intended to do when he started to walk out of the room, and additionally, in the back of my mind, I had wanted to avoid offending him by getting out of the chair as if I didn't trust him.

But I should have simply stood up and got behind the chair as he left the room. This incident made me realize that many years working in administration had indeed blunted some of my clinical instincts, and that I had much to re-learn from my workmates.

Unit staff must never second guess patient's intentions at any time and must always treat dangerous patients as if they might act in dangerous ways.

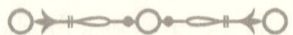

Wonderful and Weird

I have known many male patients with the diagnosis of paranoid schizophrenia who have fantasized about assaulting or killing their mothers, and some have ended up doing so. It's far more common for them to focus on their mothers than their fathers, possibly because of the emotional intensity of the mother-child bond and their inability to handle that intensity.

Sketch # 87

Mr. D. was in his early thirties, admitted on a twelve-month restoration-to-competency status, with charges of armed robbery. His psychiatric diagnoses were anxiety disorder, polysubstance abuse, and antisocial personality disorder. On the unit, he was both furtive yet also boastful and grandiose in his interactions with other patients and staff.

At the time I started psychiatric nursing in England, he would have been given the diagnosis: "inadequate psychopath," meaning someone with grand stories to tell about himself and his achievements with even grander plans for the future, while obviously lacking the wherewithal to make any of this actually happen.

He tried to hang around with a small group of younger, smarter patients, who appeared to tolerate him in case he might ever be useful to them, but who clearly saw him as not being a real peer.

One night I was doing safety checks on the patient rooms when he jumped from behind his bedroom door and stuck something against my back. He said that it was a knife that he was holding in his sweatshirt pocket, and that if I didn't help him to escape he would stab me in the neck with it.

I figured that, if he really did have a knife, he would have shown it to me to scare me. I figured that is was really his finger sticking into me. But I was alone with him in a small room, and I was certainly not going to escalate the situation at that point by challenging him on the issue, or by pressing the hospital-wide alarm that I wore around my neck. He said that I was to tell other staff members that I was taking him off the unit to get some candy from a vending machine in a corridor. When we were off the unit, I was to let him out of one of the hospital entrances on the corridor.

As soon as we were out of his room, I pressed my alarm and ran yelling toward the nursing station while he went back into his room and pretended to be asleep. A police search showed that he had no weapon.

Thoughts: This was very poorly thought out escape plan that failed for many obvious reasons. I suspect that one or two other patients may have initially agreed to take part in the attempt, or encouraged him to do it, but that when the time actually came, they figured that it had such a poor chance of success that it wasn't worth risking extra jail time for.

Forensic psychiatric nurses have to assume at all times that at least one patient is planning to escape, as probably all patients will think about it at some point in their hospitalization. Most patients know that the chances of successful escape are very slim. However, young sociopaths who are impulsive, thrill-seeking, and defiant, may think escape worth attempting simply as an adventure, or to prove their credentials to their peers.

Sketch # 88

In 2006, a new forty-two-million-dollar hospital was built, replacing the old ramshackle, overcrowded buildings. It was specifically designed as a forensic psychiatric hospital, and although the units turned out to be more problematically spacious than we had initially envisaged, it provided an outstanding environment to work in.

During one of the planning meetings, an architect comment that they had decided to have limestone slabs by the main entrance to the hospital rather than using concrete, although the latter would have been much cheaper. He explained that the rationale for this was that they wanted to create an "air of permanence" to the hospital that only real stone could provide.

In an era when many public psychiatric hospitals were closing, he hoped that the staff and the public in general would have some reassurance that the hospital would be around for a long time if it was seen to be built of stone rather than concrete.

In the state of Ohio, when a new public building is being designed, a small percentage of the total cost has to be dedicated to artwork in that building. Part of this artwork at the hospital included a series of large metal curves placed in the main dining area.

At one of the opening ceremonies of the hospital, the artist who created them explained that the concept of a psychiatric hospital being a community in itself had intrigued him. He said that it brought to his mind the mythical city of Atlantis, with his following the interpretation of the story in which Atlanteans actually survived after the island had sunk under the ocean. He then saw this Atlantis community as being made up of essentially normal people only different in some ways to those humans who lived in communities above water. Similarly, he saw the psychiatric hospital as an integrated community, only made up of people different in some ways than those in other communities.

The curved metal sculpture was intended to represent the waves on the ocean surface above Atlantis when it became submerged, to make this parallel.

Thought: When I retired, I found myself wondering who would remember this sort of trivia about the hospital. Even just a few years after the new hospital had been opened, no one could recall anything about this when I asked, and I started to think about what would become of this knowledge when the architect and artist retired or died.

I wondered if, even in our highly technological age, human memory put into writing may still have a useful place.

References

1. Szasz, T. 1974. *The Myth of Mental Illness: Foundations of a Theory of Personal Conduct.* New York: Harper and Row.
2. King, M. 2017. "Psychiatric Nursing: Medical Science or Social Science?" *British Journal of Nursing* 26 (17) September 27: 990–991.
3. King, M. 2017. Psychiatric nursing: an identity crisis? *British Journal of Mental Health Nursing* Vol 6. No 6. December: 254–255
4. King, M. 2015. "Charles Darwin and the Asylum Letters." *American Journal of Psychiatry* 172(4): 321–322.
5. Ryland, R., and M. King. 1976. "Queer Turns." *Nursing Mirror* September 2: 63–65.
6. King, M. 1981. "Dependency in Agoraphobia: A woman in Need." *Nursing Mirror* January 22: 34–36.
7. Orlando, I. 1961. *The Dynamic Nurse-Patient Relationship: Function, Process, and Principles.* New York: Putnam.
8. King, M., and R. Ryland. 1982. "An Overdose of Attitudes." *Nursing Mirror* June 9: 40–41.
9. King, M. 1982. "Look Back in Anger." *Nursing Mirror* October 20: 52–54.
10. Allen B., and D. Bosta. 2002. *Games Criminals Play*. Sacramento. Rae John.
11. King M., and R. Ryland. 1981. "Thank You, Mr. Jones, (but what do you want?)." *Nursing Mirror* 153(21): 40–41.
12. Marker, C. 1987. "The Marker Model: A Hierarchy for Nursing Standards." *Nursing Journal of Quality Assurance* 1(2).
13. Lowell, R. 1988. Selected Poems. New York: Farrar Straus and Giroux: 87-88.
14. Richards, L. 1911. *Reminiscences of Linda Richardson, America's First Trained Nurse*, Boston: Whitcomb & Barrows.
15. Stevenson, R. L. 1909. Virginibus Puerisque. London: Chatto and Windus: 35.

Author Biography

Malcolm King, RN, MS, CS, worked as a psychiatric nurse for forty-four years, in twelve hospitals, three countries, and four US states, starting as a nursing assistant and eventually becoming a director of nursing. His book, *Wonderful and Weird*, is a compilation of the clinical case studies and administrative issues that were most influential in guiding him to an understanding of the role of the psychiatric nurse and nursing administrator in providing the best possible care to their patients.

The book reviews the positive and negative impacts on psychiatric nursing practice as the theoretical models of psychiatry moved from the psychosocial-psychodynamic model to the current biological-medical model, and how those models themselves may be influenced by political trends.

The particular issues for the nurse working with a forensic psychiatry population are discussed, focusing on the need for nurses to be aware of their professional and personal boundaries with this patient group.

Wonderful and Weird will be of interest to those psychiatric nurses making decisions regarding the development of their own careers, and to both educators of psychiatric nurses and educators of general nursing students doing their dreaded psychiatric rotation.

www.ingramcontent.com/pod-product-compliance
Lightning Source LLC
Chambersburg PA
CBHW031049180526
45163CB00002BA/747